History of Ophthalmology 1

Academiae Ophthalmologicae Internationalis

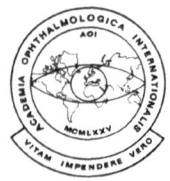

Board

President: F.C. Blodi
Vice-Presidents: P. Brégeat
                 J. Fronimopoulos
Secretary-General: A. Nakajima
Treasurer: W. Duque-Estrada

History of Ophthalmology 1

Sub auspiciis
Academiae Ophthalmologicae Internationalis

Editor H.E. HENKES
Geervliet, The Netherlands

Associate Editor Cl. ZRENNER
Munich, F.R.G.

Kluwer Academic Publishers
DORDRECHT · BOSTON · LONDON

Published by Kluwer Academic Publishers,
P.O. Box 17, 3300 AA Dordrecht, The Netherlands

Kluwer Academic Publishers incorporates the publishing programmes of D. Reidel,
Martinus Nijhoff, Dr W. Junk and MTP Press.

Sold and distributed in the U.S.A. and Canada
by Kluwer Academic Publishers,
101 Philip Drive, Norwell, MA 02061, U.S.A.

In all other countries, sold and distributed
by Kluwer Academic Publishers Group,
P.O. Box 322, 3300 AH Dordrecht, The Netherlands.

Reprinted from *Documenta Ophthalmologica*, Vol. 68, Nos. 1-2 (1988).

ISBN-13: 978-94-010-7081-2   **e-ISBN-13 : 978-94-009-1307-3**
DOI : 10.1007 / 978-94-009-1307-3

Table of contents

Documenta Ophthalmologica 68: 1 (1988)
© Kluwer Academic Publishers, Dordrecht

Introduction

With this issue of the Documenta Ophthalmologica we begin a new endeavor. The objective is to dedicate an occasional issue of the Documenta to historical topics in ophthalmology. This issue will be sponsored by the Academia Ophthalmologica Internationalis and will be edited by Professor Dr. Harold Henkes, a member of the Academia: with the historian Dr. Claudia Zrenner of Munich as Associate Editor.

The last decade has shown that interest in historical topics is on the increase. We have seen a French society dedicated to this aspect of ophthalmology. This society not only convenes annually, but also publishes a most interesting annual report. We have similarly seen the founding of a "Julius Hirschberg Society" which is directed more toward the German-speaking countries, but has an international character. The Academia Ophthalmologica Internationalis has since its inception been most interested in the history of ophthalmology. At the annual meeting a good number of excellent papers are read which deal mainly with historical topics. The quality of these papers has been so high that the Academia decided to have those published and we are grateful to Professor Henkes and the publishers of Documenta Ophthalmologica to have given us an opportunity to print these communications. These issues of Documenta should enhance further interest in the history of our specialty.

Frederick C. Blodi, M.D.
President
Academia Ophthalmologica
Internationalis

Documenta Ophthalmologica 68: 3–8 (1988)
© Kluwer Academic Publishers, Dordrecht

Four legends about Hippocrates
Collected by Mr. Zarakas of the Village Pili – Cos

J. FRONIMOPOULOS* & J. STEFANELLIS**
Neofytou Bamva St. 6, Athens 138, Greece

A number of legends about Hippocrates (Fig. 1) are still being told by and to the inhabitants of the Island of Cos.

First legend

While Hippocrates was practicing in Cos, a rich man from another place visited him. This man had been suffering from a severe illness for a long time, and had consulted many physicians, none of whom had been able to cure him. He had heard about the famous doctor Hippocrates, and in spite of the fact that he had more or less resigned himself to the fact that his illness seemed incurable, he travelled to Cos to meet Hippocrates and ask for a treatment.

Hippocrates examined him thoroughly and said, "*I recognize your illness, but, unfortunately, I do not have the means to cure you; the medicine you need is not available.*" The sick man was desperate when he heard these words and said to himself, "*Since Hippocrates, the wisest physician in the world cannot help me, I had better go to the mountain and await my death there.*" He climbed a certain mountain and stayed alone for two or three days waiting to die. But after some time, he felt hungry and thought he should come down and look for a shepherd's house where he could ask for some milk. He set out and found one almost immediately. He began to call out, but there was no answer. He approached the yard, calling continually, but there was no sign of life. Then as he look around, to his great surprise he saw a big snake with its head in a vessel of milk drinking; the rest of its body lying on the wall (Fig. 2).

The snake, startled by the stranger's presence and disturbed, brought up the swallowed milk, and quickly disappeared over the wall. The hungry sick man was desperate, took a pot from the corner, and filled it with the

* Text.
**Sketches.

4

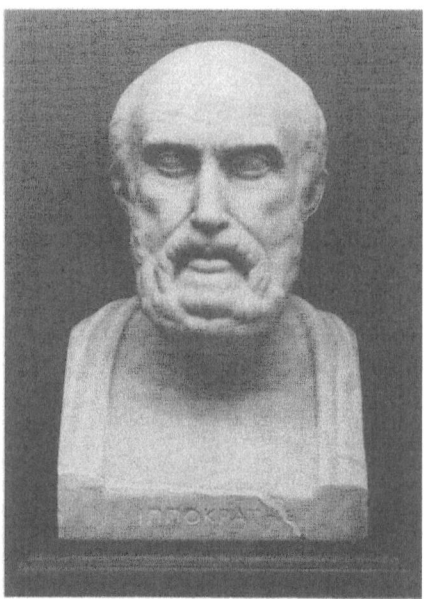

Fig. 1. Bust of Hippocrates.

poisoned milk from the vessel, saying to himself, "*Let me drink this poisoned milk, die quickly and be delivered from my torture*" (Fig. 3). Then he took the pot full of milk and returned to the mountain to drink it. Instead of being poisoned as he had believed, he felt better and continued to drink the milk. After two days he was cured. What a surprise!

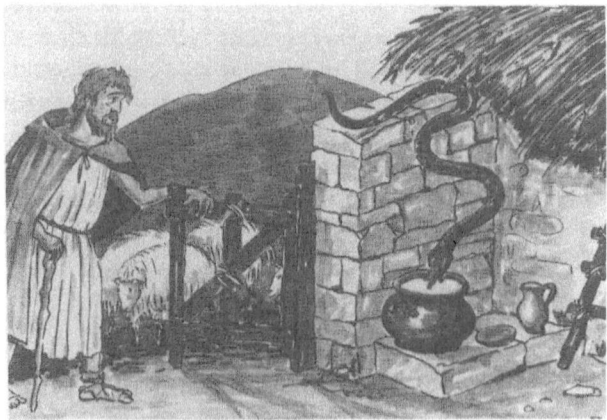

Fig. 2. The snake drinking milk.

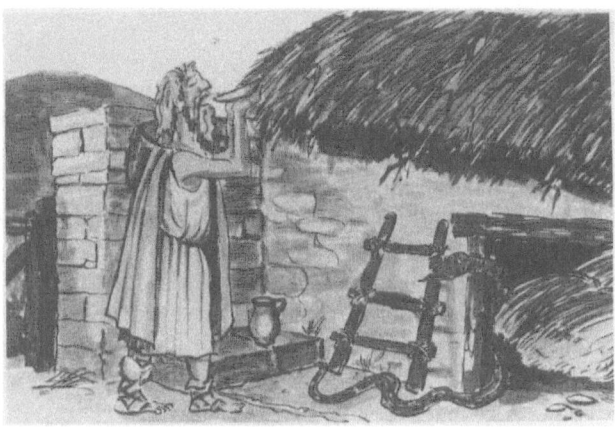

Fig. 3. The rich man drinking the poisoned milk.

Without losing any time, he hurried back to town to find Hippocrates and wanted to humiliate him as, in spite of his reputation, he had been unable to cure him.

When Hippocrates saw him, he recognized him immediately and said, "*Where did you find a seven year old snake which had drunk milk, which you also drank and thus became well again*"?

The man was amazed by Hippocrates' wisdom and admired his great knowledge of illnesses and treatments. He told him the whole story about the snake and the poisoned milk – how he drank it and was cured.

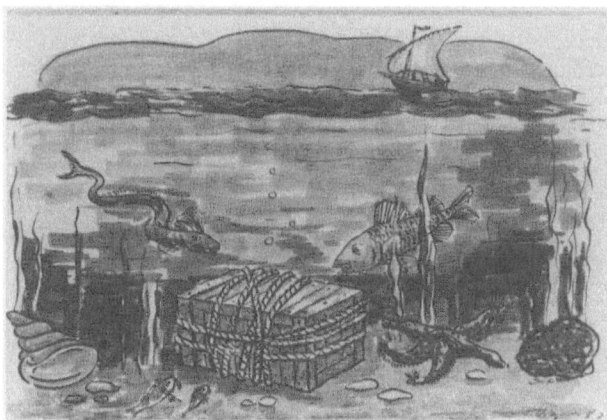

Fig. 4. The box of books sunk in the harbor of Cos.

6

Second legend

According to this legend, Hippocrates wrote about medicine in his books; put these in a marble box (Fig. 4) which he sank in Cos' harbor. But for what reason? Perhaps because people believed that these books were sacred like the Bible, and that they would be safer at the bottom of the sea where nobody would be able to find them and where they certainly would not get into the hands of barbarians, be lost or destroyed.

The Coan imagination could not conceive of a better or safer place for Hippocrates' books. Fortunately, at that time there were no deep-sea divers with oxygen masks.

Third legend

Once upon a time Hippocrates was sitting on the bank of a dry riverbed, watching two great snakes quarreling and biting each other (Fig. 5). At a certain moment one of them bit the other very severely with its poisoned fangs. Blood flowed from the great wound into the dry riverbed and the bitten snake died. Immediately water began to flow in the hitherto dry bed; the surviving snake drank the water and wet the dead snake which, in turn, revived.

Hippocrates observed this scene, rushed away to find a pot, and returning, filled it with the river water (Fig. 6). According to legend, he used this healing water to cure patients.

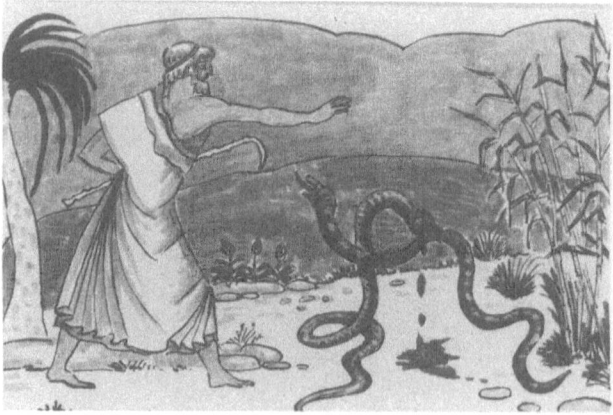

Fig. 5. Two large snakes quarreling and fighting.

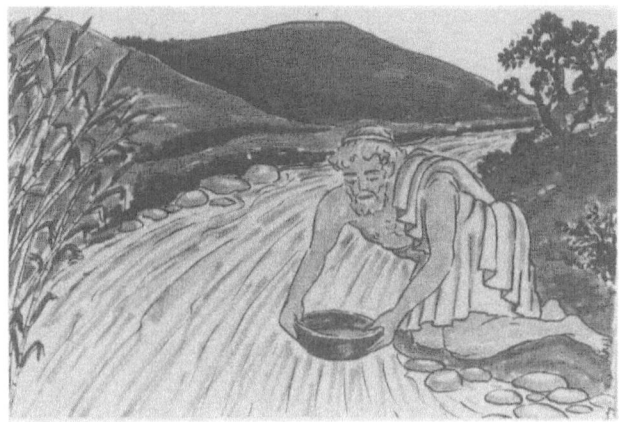

Fig. 6. Hippocrates filling a pot with the miraculous water.

The Coan imagination in this case sees Hippocrates creating "miracles" with the immortal water, enabling him to cure illness with his superhuman power.

Fourth legend

There is in existence yet another legend – this time about Hippocrates' death.

On discovering a certain herbal medicine with reviving and rejuvenating capacities, he decided to try it out first on himself before administering it to others. Thus, he took a great vessel, placed it in a hole, and put some of the medicine into it, saying to his servant. *"Cut me into small pieces and throw them into the vessel; close it and cover it well. After forty days you may come and open the vessel and you will see me revived and transformed into a baby. If anyone comes asking for me, tell them that you don't know where I am. Do not betray the secret under any circumstances – for if you open the vessel before the forty days have passed, you will find me dead."*

The servant did as Hippocrates ordered. But at that time an epidemic attacked Persia and the King sent a mission to request the help and presence of Hippocrates. Arriving at his house the messengers asked to see Hippocrates. The servant told them that he did not know where his master was. They came back again and again, asking for information and his whereabouts. Finally, the servant was unable to withhold the secret any more; they found the closed vessel and opened it (Fig. 7) – it was just at the time when Hippocrates was beginning to revive. He died because the vessel was opened

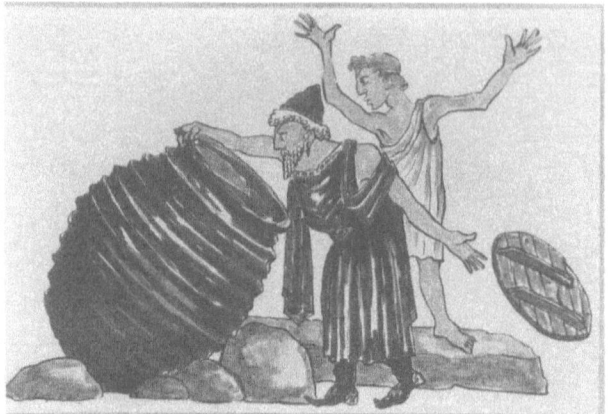

Fig. 7. The premature opening of the vessel in which Hippocrates awaited his cure.

before the forty days had passed, when the experiment would have been completed.

According to legend, people believed that Hippocrates, with his perfect knowledge, could revive men with an unknown method, but in keeping with his great humanistic and ethical ideals, he could not allow himself to experiment on others before having tried it out personally.

Comment

It is surprising how these legends, like so many others about Hippocrates' life, still circulate among the Coans; stories of the past which come to us through the mist of myth and illusion created through the ages by man's imagination.

Address for offprints: Prof. John Fronimopoulos, Neofytou Bamva St. 6, Athens 138, Greece

Documenta Ophthalmologica 68: 9–17 (1988)
© Kluwer Academic Publishers, Dordrecht – Printed in the Netherlands

Eye votives in Greek antiquity

WOLFGANG JAEGER
Mozartstr. 17a, D-6900 Heidelberg, BRD

At the museum of Cos one can find a mosaic showing the arrival of
Asklepios on this island (Fig. 1). Hippokrates is sitting on the left. On the
right, a man is standing in the foreground, greeting the god with his raised
hand. We do not know, if this is the gesture of salutation, or if it is the
gesture of a votant appealing in pain and sorrow to the god of medical art
who is still sitting in the boat.

The disorders of the eye played the most important role among the
illnesses, where one asked for the help of Asklepios. On the one hand, we
can conclude this from the number of dedicated votives. On the other hand,
we know about cures of eye-diseases in Sanctuaries of Asklepios from
numerous reports.

Unfortunately, on the isle of Cos only a few of these votives remained.
However, there is evidence that ocular votives, published as a part of private
collections in the beginning of this century, originate from Cos. In 1912, a

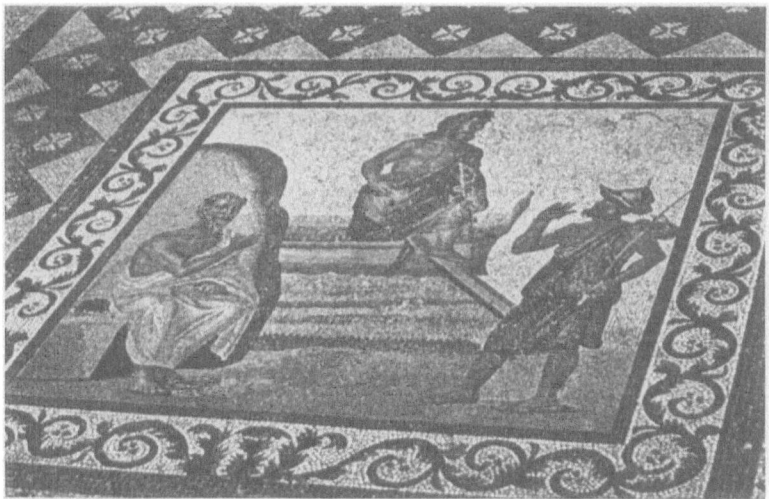

Fig. 1. Mosaic showing the arrival of Asklepios on the island of Cos (Museum of Cos) 2nd
or 3rd century A.D.

Presented at the Meeting of the Hellenic Ophthalmological History Club in Cos, 1984.

German historian of medicine [1] wrote about antique votive-gifts and demonstrated an ocular votive out of silver-plated bronze metal, originating from the temple area of the Asklepieion on Cos. Unfortunately, this piece has been lost.

We can assume that many eye-votives existed in the Asklepieion. Although there is no list of votives in Cos, there is such a catalogue for the Asklepieion in Athens [2]., from which we can learn that the number of ocular votives was the largest one amongst all votive tablets.

From such figures, however, we learn nothing about the history of the diseases leading to these dedications. It is extremely rare, that a pathological condition is shown on these eyes [3].

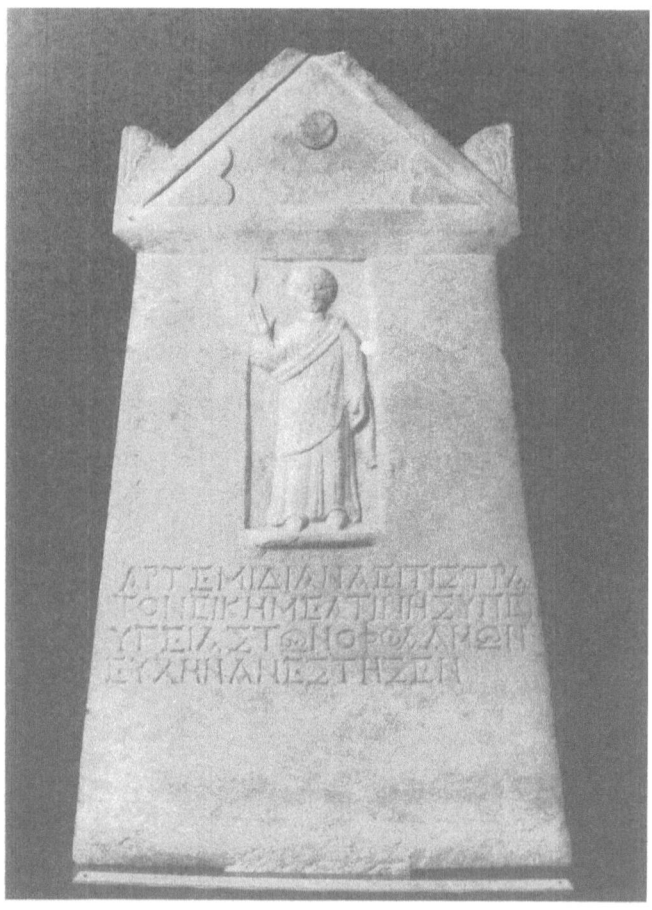

Fig. 2. Stela from Smyrna dedicated to Artemis (Museum Leyden – Inv. Nr. SNS 312).

Much more information can be drawn from the Stelae whose inscriptions give further clues. A Stela of the museum in Leyden from Smyrna (Fig. 2) is dedicated not to Asklepios but to Artemis. The votant had dedicated it "hyper hygieias ton ophthalmon" [4].

Inscriptions from the Asklepieion in Epidaurus give more detailed information [5]. Following an inscription in Epidaurus, for example, the vision of Ambrosia from Athens, who lost her sight unilaterally, was restored. The text of the inscription is as follows: "Ambrosia appealed for help to the god. Walking around in the sanctuary, she laughed at some of the stories of healing as unbelievable. She thought that it would be impossible that crippled and blind sufferers recuperated after having dreamed in the sanctuary. But while sleeping in the temple she had a dream. It seemed to her as if the god came to her and said, that he would restore her to health, but that she would have to devote a silver-pig to the temple as a fee and remembrance of her foolishness. After these words the god had scratched her sick eye with a knife and instilled a remedy into the eye. At dawn, she left the sanctuary in perfect health."

In this story no eye-votive, but a silver-pig was set up as sign of thanks for sucessful healing. We can account, however, that the usual *reward for successful healing* was the dedicating of a copy of that organ, that was cured and among all organs the eye is the one most suited for such images.

Another group of votives was offered in the *search for help*. This is apparent from inscriptions, which are combined with the votives [6].

Finally, in Greek mythology we find one other reason for dedicating such votives – a reason which is not to be found in the later christian world: there exist examples where gods impose *eye diseases as punishment,* if men failed to keep a promise. For example, a man named Diogenes set up a monument with an inscription that he had failed to keep a vow concerning the healing of sick cattle. The gods imposed an eye-disease on his daughter. Together with his daughter he devoted a monument as a compensation [7].

Among the votives of the eye only material such as terra-cotta, stone and metal is preserved. It is likely that wooden or wax – votives which existed as offerings of the poorer population, are no longer existing. Also, votives in precious metal are only exceptionally to be found. In most cases even insets of the iris and pupil, mostly manufactured out of precious metal, have been broken out of the eyes. In most ocular images from Delphi [8] the iris and pupils are missing. Only if there were no insets and if the iris and pupil probably painted on – like in a 14 cm large colossal marble eye – the entire eye has been preserved.

The most simple and inexpensive material was terra-cotta. The three examples of Fig. 3 originate from the Asklepieion of Corinth [9]. The eye

12

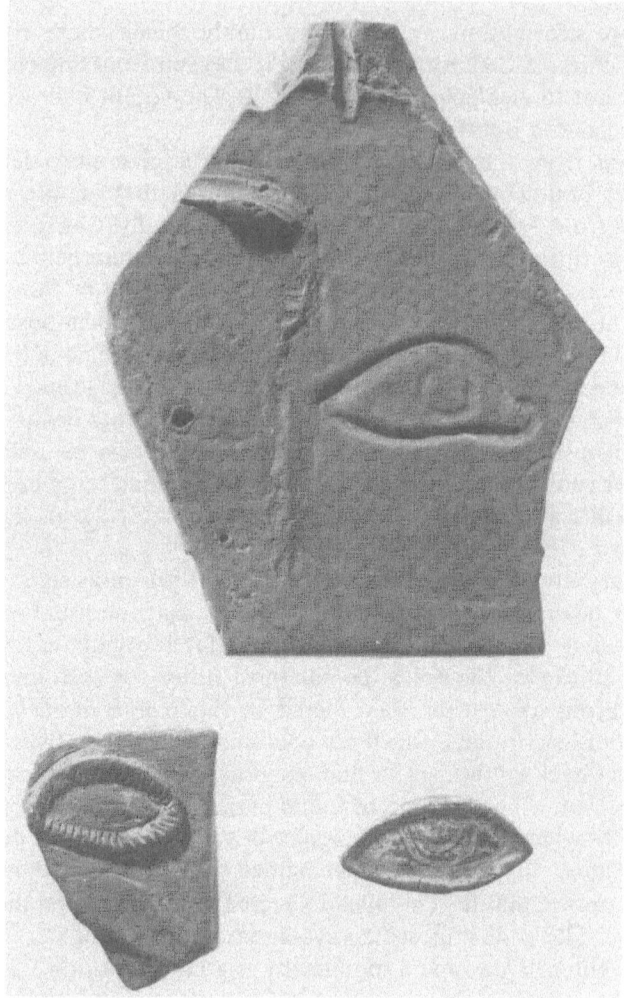

Fig. 3. Eye-votives in terra-cotta, found in the Asklepieion of Corinth (Nrs. 13, 14 and 15. Publ. R. Roebuck).

could be scratched or worked as relief before firing the terra-cotta. The eyelashes are made in a simple way. Furthermore, this material had the advantange that additionally an inscription could be engraved, like in a votive from Cyprus [10], which is unfortunately only preserved as a drawing (Fig. 4). The inscription shows, that besides Asklepios also a number of other gods have been invoked. In this case it is Theos Hypsistos. But also Apollo and Artemis, Demeter and Hagne Aphrodite were known for healing eye diseases as well as Serapis, Isis and Anoubis, the Egyptian gods infiltrat-

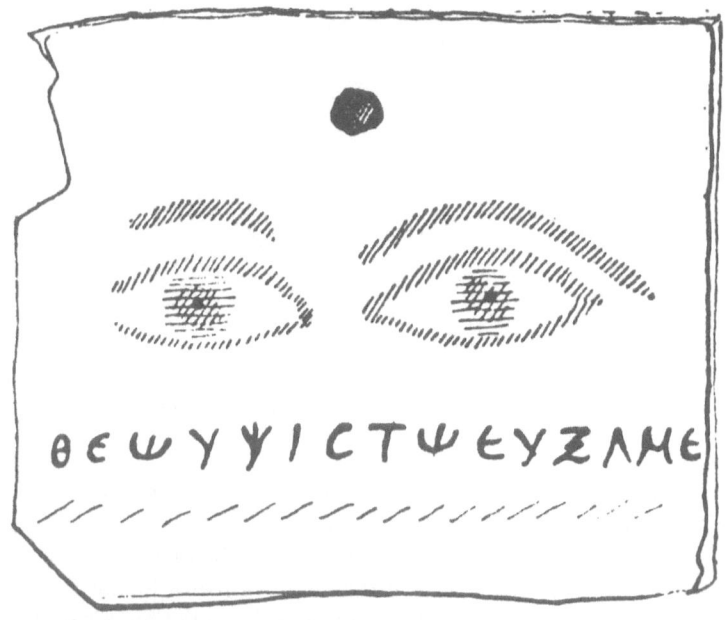

Fig. 4. Eye-votive from Cyprus, dedicated to the "Theos hypsistos".

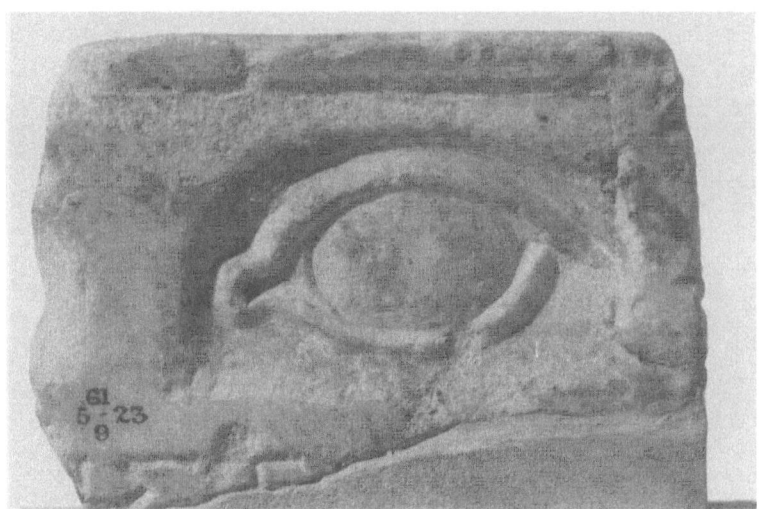

Fig. 5. Fragment of a votive relief representing a pair of eyes. Dedicated to "(Zeus) the most high". Presented in 1861 by the 5th Earl of Aberdeen to the British Museum (Reproduced by courtesy of the trustees of the British Museum, London – Arch. Nr. 802).

14

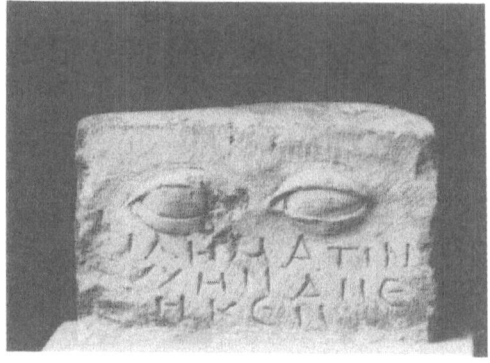

Fig. 6. Votive tablet with relief representing a pair of eyes with inscription. Pnyx Athens. Elgin collection (British Museum, London – Arch. Nr. 801).

ing the greek world in this period. The most common dedications, however, were addressed to Asklepios.

The following ocular votives of marble came from the Asklepieion in Athens [10] and came together with the Elgin-Marbles to the British Museum in London. Fig. 5 shows a fragment of votive relief representing a pair

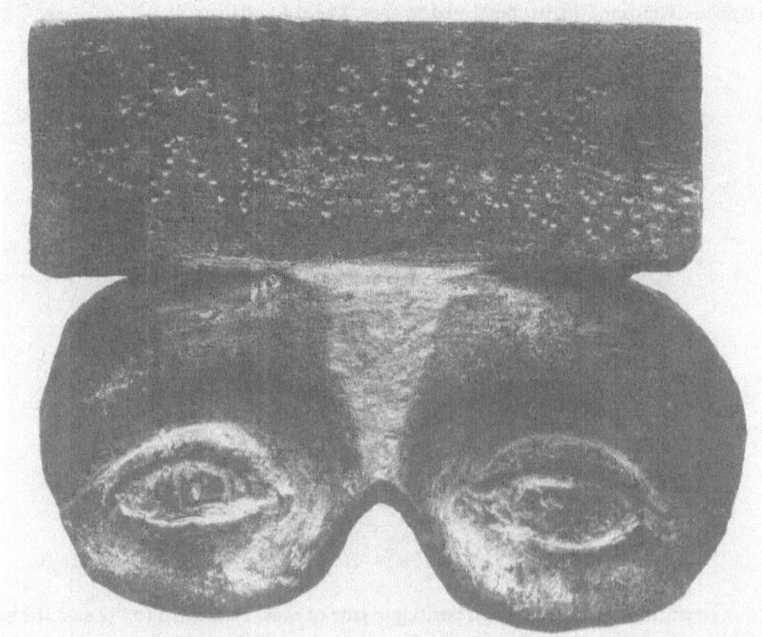

Fig. 7. Pair of eyes found in Pergamon. A votive with inscription in dotted letters. (Inv. Nr. Mb, 1959, M3.)

of eyes, of which the iris and pupil were probably painted. Fig. 6 demonstrates a pair of eyes with inscription that mentioned the name of the votant.

Besides those examples of single and double eyes *ocular images resembling a mask* exist in Greek antiquity. Not only the rim of eyelids with eyelashes, but also the eyebrows together with a part of the forehead are shown. The ocular votives of this kind found so far are made out of bronze.

The pair of eyes shown in Fig. 7 has been found in Pergamon [12]. The name of the donor is inscribed in the rectangular tablet in dotted writing.

An even more beautiful bronze ocular votive (Fig. 8) has been found in the lower town of Herakleia. The actual name of this South-Italian town is Policoro [13]. Close to the place of discovery of this votive a chapel of St. Lucia is situated [14], who is, since early christianity, the most important saint helping in ocular diseases. Also in this chapel eye votives are to be found and it is most impressive to see a tradition in the same place surviving over centuries and during all tempests that have gone over this country.

St. Lucia is celebrated in the catholic church in Italy and Spain on the 13th of December. On the same day St. Ottilie is celebrated in Germany, Austria and France, that means that she takes the place of St. Lucia in this area as the special saint for eye disorders [15].

Also the orthodox church has a special saint for eye diseases. It is St. Paraschevi, whose celebration day is also the 13th of December. There exists a Paraschevi chapel of the Johanniter-castle in Cos. Also in the main church of Cos icons of St. Paraschevi are found, which are decorated with many eye votives.

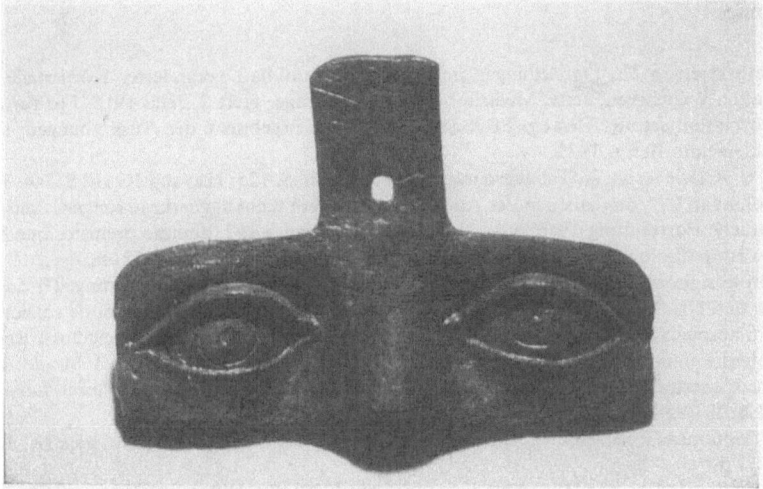

Fig. 8. Eye votive found in Herakleia (Policoro). (Courtesy of Prof. B. Neutsch.)

16

Such eye votives are dedicated up to the present time. They indicate that patients on one hand hope to be cured by the techniques of modern medicine, on the other hand, however, they ask for help trusting with all their faith in celestial powers. If one compares these christian votives with votives of Greek antiquity, one can see that these testimonies of faith, of hope and of thankfulness have not changed in the last 2000 years.

Acknowledgements

I want to express my thanks to the following museums, from which I got photographs for publication: The British Museum, London WC 1B 3DG, Dept. of Greek and Roman Antiquities; Corinth Excavations, American School of Classical Studies, 54 Soudias Str., Athens 140 (Mrs. Nancy Bookidis); Deutsches Archäologisches Institut Instanbul, Taksim Sira Selvi (Dr. W. Radt); Rijksmuseum van Oudheden, Rapenburg 28, 2311 EW Leiden (Prof. F.L. Bastet).

Moreover, I want to thank Prof. A. Dihle and Prof. F. Gschnitzer, who were always helpful in finding examples of eye-votives in the literature. From Prof. B. Neutsch I got the photograph of the wonderful eye-votive of Herakleia. I am especially thankful to him for his remarks about the continuity of eye-votives in Greek antiquity, in the medieval period and in modern times.

References

1. Meyer-Steineg Th. Darstellungen normaler und krankhaft veränderter Körperteile an antiken Weihgaben. Jena, Medizin-historische Beiträge. Heft 2, Jena 1912. For further information see: R. Herzog, I.P. Schazmann, Kos, Ergebnisse der Ausgrabungen. Das Asklepieion. Berlin 1932.
2. IG II². Clasis tertia. A. Tabulae curatorum aesculapii. S. 125–128: and IG II². S. 344–345.
3. Frohmann C. Votivgaben in der Antike, insbesondere bei Augenerkrankungen. Zeitschr ärztliche Fortbildung 1956; 50: 133–135; and F. Regnault: L'homme préhistorique Les ex-voto pathologiques romains. in: L'Homme Préhistorique 1910; 8: 321–336.
4. Corpus signorum classicorum Leyden 1982. Eds. F.L. Bastet and H. Brunsting. Tb. 56 Nr 206 (inv Nr. SNs 312). Other references about this Stela: Tituli Asiae minoris collecti et editi auspiciis academiae litterarum austriacae. Vol. V Tituli Lydiae, Fasciculus I Regio septentrionalis and orientem vergens. Ed. J. Keil and P. Herrmann, Vienna 1981 and: The Greek inscriptions in the Rijksmuseum van Oudheden at Leyden by H.W. Pleket, Leyden, E.J Brill, 1958.
5. Inscriptiones Graecae IV. 2. Auf. Fasz 1 (Berlin 1929). Ed. Hiller v. Gaertringen Nr. 121, Z. 33 ff.
6. Inscriptiones Graecae IV. 2. Aufl. Fasz. 1 (Berlin 1929). Ed. Hiller v. Gaertringen Nr. 121, Z. 72 ff and Z. 125 f.

7. Exploration Archéologique de Délos. Le mobilier délien par W. Deonna. Paris E. de Boccard, Editeur, 1938; 215–220. and: P. Herrmann: Ergebnisse einer Reise in Nordost-Lydien. Denkschrift des Archäologischen Institutes Wien, 1962; 80: 45–57.

8. Fouilles de Delphes Bd. V, Fasz. 1, Ed. P. Perdrizet, D. 208–209, Paris 1908.

9. Corinth. Results of Excavations conducted by the American School of Classical Studies at Athens. Vol. XIV. The Asklepieion and Lerna by: Carl Roebuck. The American School of Classical Studies at Athens, Princetown, New Jersey, 1951; 120–122.

10. L.P. de Cesnola, Cypern, seine alten Städte, Gräber und Tempel. Dt Ausgabe Jena 1879; 129 and 361–362.

11. IG II². Donaria reliquorum deorum et Heroum. S. 307. Nr. 4799 and 4805

12. Altertümer von Pergamon (Deutsches Archäologisches Institut. Herausgegeben im Auftrage des Instituts von Erich Boehringer. Bd. VIII 3. Die Inschriften des Asklepieions. von Christian Habicht. Walter de Gruyter & Co., Berlin 1969; 117, and 127–128.

13. Neutsch B. Grabungen und Funde in Apulien und Lukanien von 1950–1965. Archäologischer Anzeiger, Beiblatt zum Jahrbuch des Deutschen Archäologischen Instituts, Bd. 81, 1966. Walter de Gruyter & Co., Berlin, 1966/67, S. 297–300.

14. Personal communication of B. Neutsch.

15. Jaeger W. Augenvotive. Thorbecke-Verlag, Sigmaringen. 1979.

Documenta Ophthalmologica 68: 19–34 (1988)
© Kluwer Academic Publishers, Dordrecht

Leonardo and the eye

ROBERT WEALE
*Department of Visual Science, Institute of Ophthalmology, University of London, Judd St.,
London WC1H 9QS, UK*

Introduction

It is curious that the many facets of Leonardo's Notebooks that have been
studied have excluded what he had to say about the eye. True, Keele (1980),
in his monumental work on the artist's anatomical drawings kept at Windsor, deals with some ophthalmic points. But, understandably, he has not
sought out what might be of interest to eye and vision specialists, and so
missed information that sheds light not only on Leonardo's own eyes, but
also on aspects of his painting which may be of interest to historians of art.

There are entries in Leonardo's notes which leave one perplexed. How is
it that the man who was the first to draw and to understand the nature of
interference in wave-motion should have been ignorant about refraction?
Why did a mind that taught us to base observation on controlled experiment
become so obsessed with the optical anomalies attendant on vision through
a pin-hole as to fail to devise the simplest of tests disproving that image-size
depends on illumination?

Of course, one's comments have to be guarded: ignorance may more
readily be found in the reader's mind than in that of the writer. We have to
try and forget that we are children of our own time and to see Leonardo in
his own right: this implies that his experimental work has to be judged on
its merits without even a whiff of hindsight. However, insofar as the laws of
reasoning and logic have not appreciably changed over the last five centuries, we should be allowed to assess the validity of his conclusions and
beliefs.

His understanding of refraction

Leonardo was occupied with both optical and visual questions, and it is
arguable that, in his days, the distinction between the two was tenuous.
Optical instruments were unknown – more than a century was to elapse

before Galileo would invent his eponymous telescope – and simple lenses were crude with image construction as yet not comprehended. The paradox of Leonardo being the first person to have understood and drawn the course of rays before and after reflection from a concave surface such as the inside of a tea-cup, yet to have drawn rays passing unbent through a glass of water (Fig. 1), is easy to resolve. He saw a parallel between reflexion and the collision between a ball and a wall, and correctly spelled out the laws of reflexion on the basis of the mechanical paradigm (Fig. 2) without necessarily grasping the principles of optics.

His drawing of refraction is incomprehensible for three reasons. In the first place, he knew that light is bent on passing from a less dense into a denser medium: e.g. when discussing the use of presbyopic (reading) glasses (MSG 90a), he mentions a straight line [i.e. a ray] being bent during passage through the lens. He also appreciated that a virtual image is formed (see p. 32). Secondly, the laws of refraction were not undiscovered at the time of the Renaissance. More than a millenium earlier, Ptolemy had discovered a relation between angles of incidence and refraction which resembled Snell's Law at least for small angles, an approximation whereon simple image construction is based even to-day. But Leonardo does not seem to have come across it, even though he had read Witelo's work on optics.

And thirdly, he was aware that the cornea refracts light. He showed more than once that what he called the central line was undeviated (Fig. 3), with the rest fanning out. It remains to be demonstrated, however, that this followed from a real grasp of refraction: remember that, early on, he was wedded to the emissive hypothesis of vision, according to which the visual spirit of an image emanated from the eye (Codex Atlanticus 90 r.b). But once

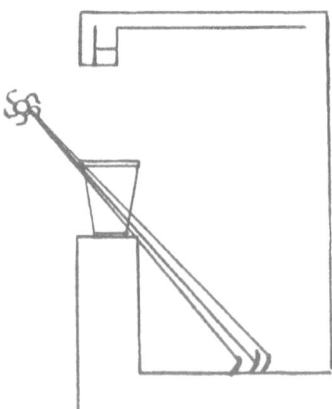

Fig. 1. Illustration of rainbow colours produced by a glass of water (Windsor [Leoni] 145; Ab).

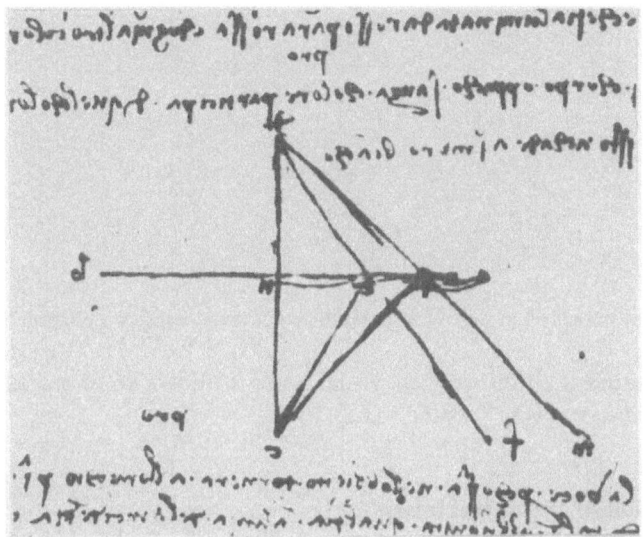

Fig. 2. The laws of reflexion (MS A de l'Institut, 19 v.).

he had observed that displacement of one of his eye-balls, gripped between two fingers, moved the image of a seen object in relation to that seen by the stationary eye, he realised that rays travel in the direction opposite to what he had assumed originally (Codex Atlanticus 227 r.a).

Another potential handicap was that Leonardo does not seem to have been acquainted with elementary trigonometry. Not only is there not to be found any trace of it in his extensive geometrical studies, but the conclusion has also to be reached from his experiments on perspective, where one faces another paradox. He clearly apprehended that his visual pyramid with its apex at the eye represented a system of projective geometry. Yet he separated projections in the vertical (image) plane from those on the horizontal planes, even though Cellini credits him with having discovered a sort of visual sphere with the eye at its centre (see also Codex Trivulzianus F29 v. 28).

Visual acuity across the visual field

It is of great ophthalmological interest that Leonardo stressed that the central ray was seen more sharply than any other (Windsor 115 r.A). He had discovered the reduction in visual acuity in the periphery of the visual field. Intuitively also he had grasped that one of the advantages of the cornea is

22

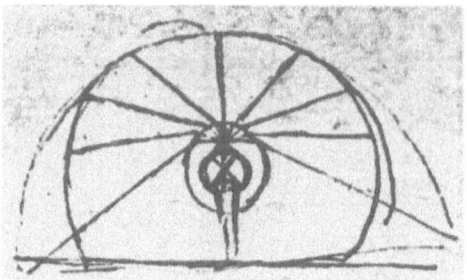

Fig. 3. Corneal refraction in the outer circle indicating the visual field (Windsor 19152 r.).

that it enhances the limits of our visual field; it allows us to see out of the corner of the eye, even "behind" (Fig. 3).

The formation of the retinal image

Leonardo's failure to understand refraction did not prevent him from attempting to describe the passage of rays inside the eye. As we shall see below, he had observed that a pinhole produces inverted images, an observation which had inspired him to the discovery of the camera obscura (Fig. 4). He concluded from this that a similar inversion must occur in the pupillary plane, as he saw no essential difference between a pupil and a pinhole. But at this stage he encountered a seemingly insuperable problem, namely that we do not see the world upside down. This paradox was resolved more than two centuries after Leonardo by Bishop Berkeley, but in the meantime Leonardo postulated a second inversion in the crystalline lens to overcome the first.

Here we find another, anatomical, problem. Whenever Leonardo drew the human crystalline lens (Fig. 5), he rendered it as a sphere. There is no immediate explanation for this. No mammalian lens is spherical; birds, sauripsidians, and fish have spherical lenses, but Leonardo's expression for lens was "spera crisstalljna" or the crystalline sphere (Windsor F118 v. A). Leonardo was no stranger to dissection: he had dissected skulls, and, indeed,

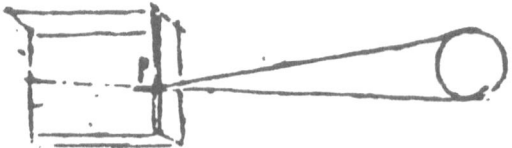

Fig. 4. Camera obscura (MS A de l'Institut 21 r.).

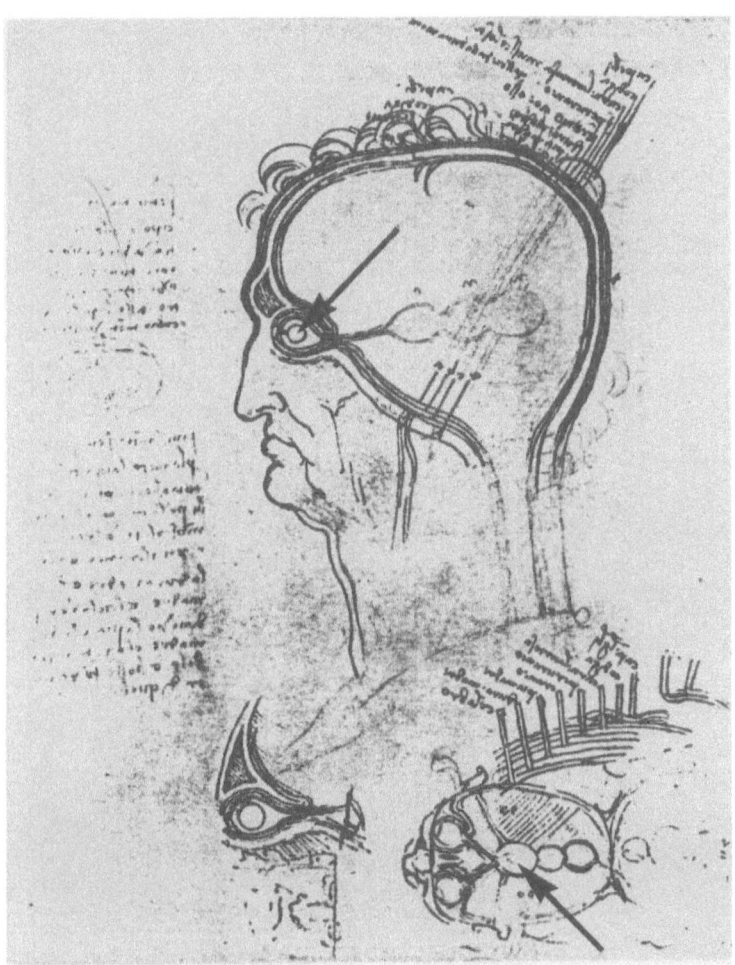

Fig. 5. Vertical sections through the scalp and the eye with the spherical lens (✓). Also a horizontal section showing three cerebral ventricles, the anterior being marked ↖ (Windsor 12603 r.).

was the first to mention and to describe the frontal sinus, presumably a reason why he used to render the overlying part of the forehead with some emphasis. It is true that he was mistaken about the course of the optic nerve though he was aware of the optic chiasma (Fig. 6); he associated the anterior ventricle (Fig. 5) with a general type of sensorium which he dubbed the imprensiva, will and memory being located in the middle and posterior ventricles respectively. Rationalisation rather than observation persuaded him that the optic nerves led to the imprensiva.

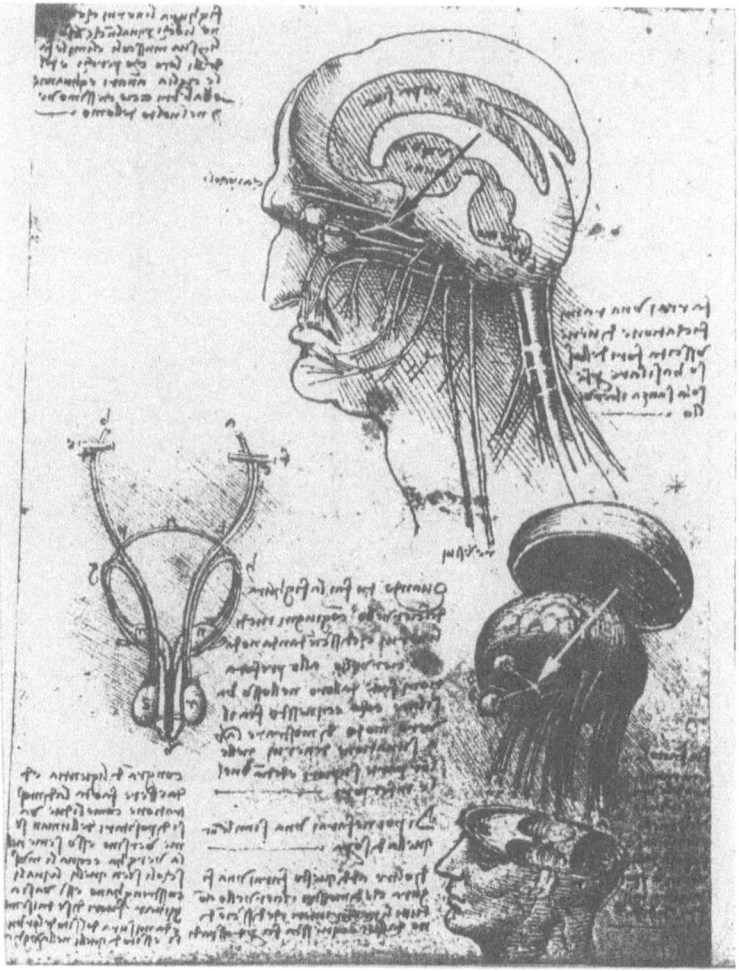

Fig. 6. The central nervous system, with the optic chiasma marked (Weimar v.).

Perhaps he found the dissection of the brain easier than that of the eye. He describes how he used a saw to open the skull: thereafter the material to deal with is soft. The human sclera calls for a sharp knife if not also for skill: but the fact is that Leonardo knew the eye to contain a lens, and it cannot be imagined that he had not actually seen one. In any case, if he had, indeed, failed to incise the sclera, surely he would have managed to extrude the lens through the pupil. I think the explanation for his gross misrepresentation is to be found in his ignorance of optics. He saw the function of the lens not as a refracting device but as one of reflexion. The pupil inverts the image,

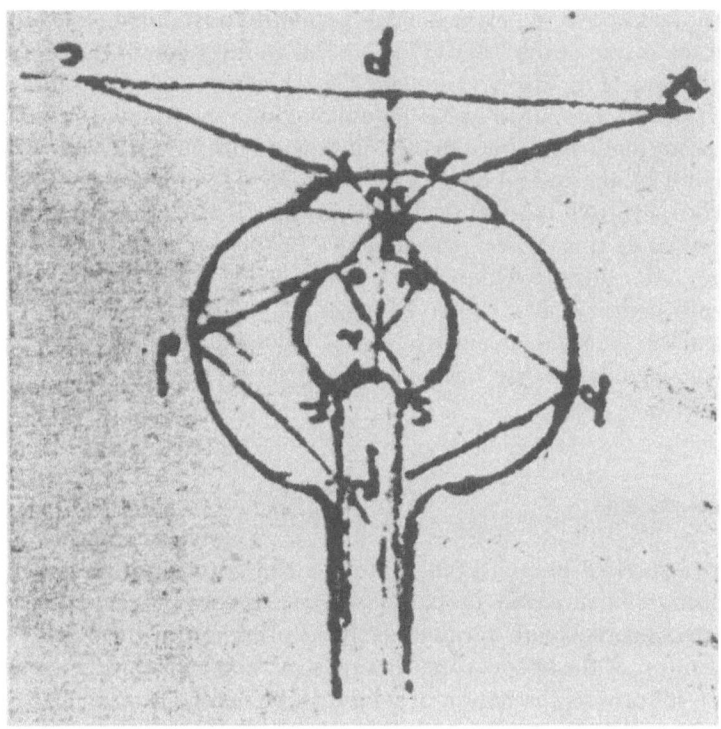

Fig. 7a. The trajectories of central and peripheral rays from an object A, b, c to the optic nerve h (MS D 10 r.).

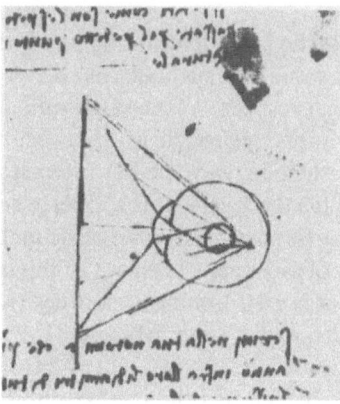

Fig. 7b. Illustration of corneal refraction and double inversion of the rays striking the optic nerve (Codex Atlant. F. 345 v. b).

as mentioned above. To make it erect, Leonardo postulated reflexion of the rays on the inside of the sclera (Fig. 7a) and an inversion of the central rays inside the lens (Fig. 7b). The imagined combination of central and peripheral rays proves Leonardo's utter failure of comprehension in these matters.

The point made here is not that Leonardo did not come to understand the production of the retinal image. In a way he was quite logical; the pupil might (be pictured to) invert the image: positive lenses clearly did the same. Hence two inverting devices in series could produce the erect images that we perceive. After all, the relevant optics was elucidated by Gauss only in the eighteenth century. But Leonardo's mental picture of how the image is formed in the eye led to an outright denial of what he must have seen, a point on which mediaeval man had clearly not yet yielded to the man of the Renaissance.

The stars mislead

Leonardo showed himself keenly interested in perception in general, and introspective phenomena in particular. He was clearly a painter, and therefore concerned with the internal effects produced by the outside world. His invention of the above word "imprensiva" confirms this by the manner in which it conveys the notion of intake and of prehension.

While he was acutely aware of objective phenomena due to light, e.g. he discovered pupillary constriction following illumination of the eye, and may be said to have realised that there existed something like a reflex, he was also anxious to render descriptions of entoptic phenomena reliable and convincing.

Leonardo was amongst the first great minds to see the value of numerical statements, but it cannot come as a surprise that he was slow to develop any appreciable deftness in that respect. At the same time he displayed considerable sophistication e.g. in his approach to as difficult a subject as photometry. It is remarkable that, in view of his interest in both this and the geometry of perspective, the discovery of the inverse square law eluded him.

The reason for this may be sought in some basic lack of understanding he had about the brightness of an image. The root of the trouble was as follows. He observed the apparent size of luminous sources through artifical pupils of varying aperture; and noted (Codex Madrid II, 25 v.) that

"the cornea of that eye which has the largest pupil will see objects more enlarged . . . An example of what has been said above presents itself when one of the major stars is seen through a small aperture in a paper placed near the pupil of the eye: you will see that star much smaller. And this occurs because the entire pupil was not used; it has been used by as much less than its entirety as the star became smaller than it appeared before. And this is not because such a hole cuts out from the eye-sight part of the observed star, since through the hole passes not only the likeness [spetie] of the star, but also a great part of the sky which surrounds it".

There are two fundamental logical errors made by Leonardo in this important topic. He failed to see that his observation was true only of point sources like stars. If the pupil aperture as such had been the overriding factor then he should have been able to make a similar observation of faces, houses, trees, and the moon. But, though he could have tested his conclusion, he failed to do so. Secondly, he failed to see that, if the apparent size of objects varies with pupil size, so should the distance between any two of them. In a variant of the camera obscura, he tested the relation between aperture and image brightness, but no displacement of the images is shown because none occurred.

Leonardo was fully aware that the shape of the aperture does not affect the size of the image (Codex Madrid II, 25 r.):

"One wonders whether, when the said pupil is long in shape, round or spherical [sic], objects appear long or round to it. Let us say by way of proof that as many are the distances of the spherical objects [from the eye] so are the forms in which such a spherical object appears to the eye . . . It makes no difference to the eye to have a cornea which is more squarish or elongated than round, in that the power of receiving the image of the external objects is equally distributed across the surface of the cornea. To prove this, let us observe an object through eyelids almost closed. The shape of the cornea will almost be in the form reproduced here (Fig. 8) and does not affect the figure of the object perceived, except for its clarity and brightness which are diminished".

This observation and conclusion are valid, but demolish what Leonardo had said on the relation between object size and pupil aperture, and what he had dwelt on time and again with emphasis and tedium.

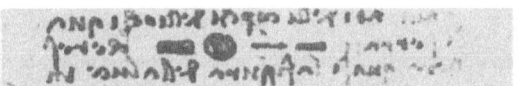

Fig. 8. The shape of the pupil depending on whether the lids are open or closing to different degrees (Codex Madrid II 25 r.).

28

It is unlikely that Leonardo would have understood that the apparent size of a point source varies with luminance because ocular irregularities scatter the light, the latter becoming subthreshold when the luminance drops too far. That said, it is also certain that Leonardo was aware of what was later to be called retinal irradiation, i.e. one of the factors linking luminance and apparent size. On more than one occasion did he draw attention to the fact that the apparent size of an object depended on the relation between its brightness and that of the background which it is seen against. In this context (Fig. 9) he demonstrated his grasp of the idea of a controlled experiment:

"Light objects against a dark background appear larger than they really are, while dark ones, on a light background, appear smaller.
The first proposition is clearly seen in the case of an iron rod of uniform thickness, of which a part has been heated to incandescence. Its former uniformity will be greatly altered, because the red-hot part will appear much thicker than the part left dark.
The second part of the proposition will be confirmed when an intersecting cold iron rod is placed between the eye and the afore-mentioned red-hot

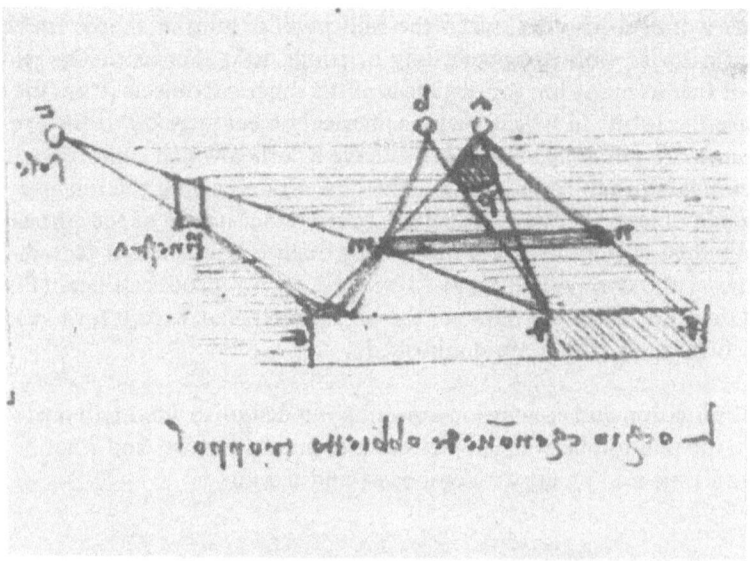

Fig. 9. To illustrate the difference in apparent thickness of glowing and cool sections of an iron rod as seen by the eyes A and b, and how this depends on the background illumination, full light being provided by "sole" passing through "finestra" (Codex Madrid II 28 v.).

iron. The cold iron will appear much thinner when juxtaposed to the hot iron, although they are of the same thickness. (And this occurs because the spirits of the visual power become overwhelmed by excess of light; they contract all their ducts in front of the light or part of it, at whichever site of the light.) Where such contraction occurs, there the objects are seen with lesser intensity and of smaller size than elsewhere".

Once again, lower luminance means smaller size.

Vision with two eyes

But the mistaken idea regarding the relation between pupil and image size led to further problems, notably in connection with binocular vision. Leonardo had demonstrated his insight into how the two eyes work conjointly by virtue of his explanation of physiological diplopia, which he not only described but also explained (Fig. 10) in terms adequate also from a present-day point of view. Incidentally, his notion of the central ray of the eye – which combined the ideas of optic axis (p. 25) with the line of optimum visual acuity (p. 22) – put the idea of fixation on a firm anatomical basis. It will be recalled that visual fixation as such was not a discovery of Leonardo's, but may more properly be attributed to Brunelleschi (1415).

The above-mentioned erroneous notion led him to a belief that he could have tested, namely (Codex Madrid II, 25 v.)

"a light seen with one eye is half as powerful and large [magnitudine] as a light seen with both eyes. Proof: let a be the imprensiva, where the eye perceives luminous objects. I affirm (Fig. 11) that b lights by only one degree of light this imprensiva. Adding b [c?] such an imprensiva receives

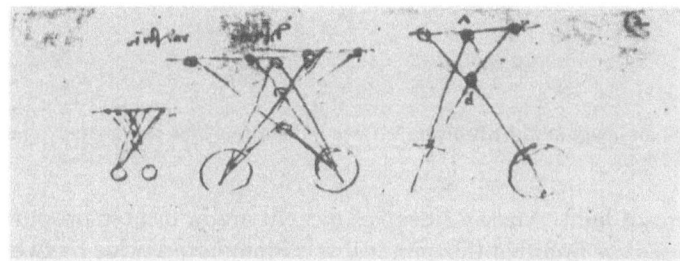

Fig. 10. The explanation of physiological diplopia [which is given in several places] (MS A de l'Institut 2 r.).

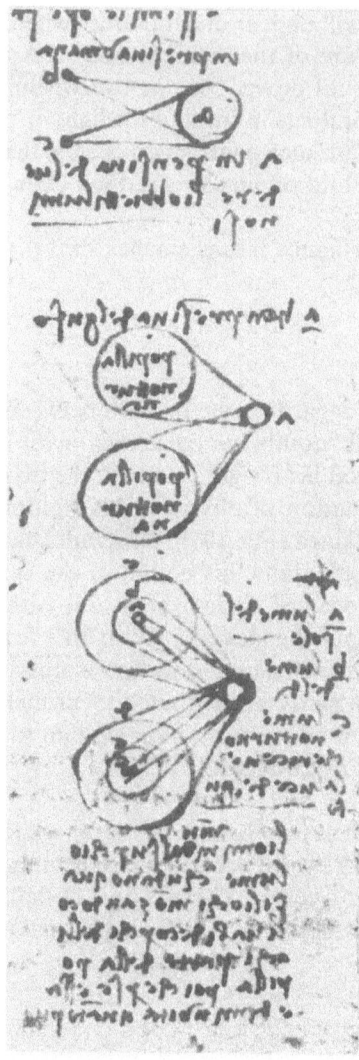

Fig. 11. Why an image seen by two eyes is twice as bright as that seen by only one (Codex Madrid II 25 v.).

2 degrees of light. And as 2 degrees of light are in double proportion to one degree, we find that the imprensiva is illuminated twice by two lights, and if it were a hundred lights, a hundred times more".

In no way will a light seen binocularly appear twice as bright as in monocular vision. But in order to understand how Leonardo arrived at this, one has to return to the camera obscura which he seems to have imagined as an analogue of the imprensiva.

He wrote (Codex Madrid II, 24 v.)

"Square cdef (Fig. 12) shall be constructed, like a room closed from all sides. On which a peep-hole will be first opened. This will illuminate the entire wall cd by one degree of light. Afterwards peep-hole b will be made, which will double the quantity of light on the afore-said wall cd, because it has acquired a second degree of light in addition to the first one".

Here there is a valid photometric argument provided the two light fluxes are superposed on the wall facing the apertures. What is not valid is likening the imprensiva to the wall: in fact, the analogy ought to have persuaded Leonardo that the two eyes do not add their responses in the way in which he had imagined it, and that his idea of imprensival function was untenable.

Presbyopia

When Leonardo was writing his Notebooks there was nothing new in senescence creating visual problems. Cicero had been well aware of some of the difficulties, and reading glasses had been known centuries before Leonardo's time: apparently they had been invented late in the thirteenth century in what, today, we call Yugoslavia (Dugački, 1977). But Leonardo attempted to elucidate the underlying mechanism:

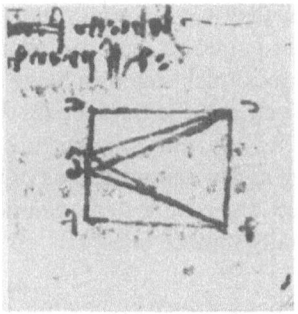

Fig. 12. The illuminance of the wall cf is one or two degrees depending on whether light passes through one aperture (A) or two (A and b) (Codex Madrid II 24 v).

"Sight is better from a distance than near in those men who are advanced in age, because the same object transmits a smaller impression of itself to the eye when it is distant than when it is near".

To begin with it is hard to interpret this. But it makes sense when one recalls Leonardo's idea of the central ray. He seems to be saying, quite validly, that a small object, if looked at, will be imaged entirely in close propinquity of the central ray, i.e. in the fovea where vision is at its most acute. He has identified a failure of the eye to resolve an image with its inability to focus it, and, incidentally, did not recall that, if we wish to see something in detail, we hold it near to our eyes (but see below).

It is clear that Leonardo knew of reading glasses, and probable that he wore a pair. He attempted to explain their function, and one has to remember that, since he did not really understand refraction, he would not have known what a focus was, not even in connection with positive lenses where it is easier to demonstrate than is true of negative ones. Note that he looks on presbyopic glasses more as a prismatic device than an imaging one:

"A proof of the manner in which glasses aid the sight: let ab (Fig. 13) be the glasses and cd the eyes, and suppose these to have grown old [invechiati]. Whereas they used to see an object at e with great ease by turning their position very considerably from the line of the optic nerves, but now by reason of age the power of bending has become weakened, and consequently it cannot be twisted without causing great pain to the eyes, so that they are constrained of necessity to place the object farther away, that is from e to f, and so see it better but not in detail. But through the interposition of the spectacles the object is clearly discerned at the distance that it was when they were young, that is at e, and this comes about because the object e passes to the eye through various media [per uario mezo], namely thin and thick, the thin being the air that is between the spectacles and the object, and the thick being the glass thickness, and so the straight line e[c] bends at ac in passing through the glass, and the object e is seen as if it were at f, without the axis of the eye having to bend away from its optic nerves; objects are then seen near at hand and better at e than at f, and especially minute ones".

It may be emphasised that Leonardo see presbyopic glasses as a magnifying instrument – which has indubitably incurred for him the opprobrium of all opticians or optometrists – and also as an anti-convergence device: it is the turning of the eyes that glasses help to avoid.

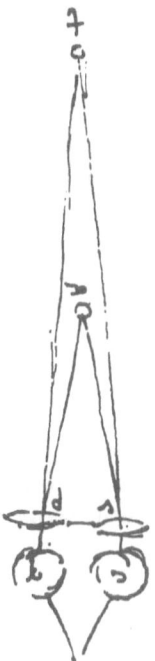

Fig. 13. How reading glasses assist the vision of the elderly (Ms G. 90a).

Conclusion

Sir Ernst Gombrich said that there are passages in Leonardo's Notebooks which are beyond our understanding. Perhaps the above comments on what Leonardo wrote on ocular anatomy and visual physiology are mistaken. While I can follow Leonardo's Italian, I cannot claim to be able to decypher all he has written even though sample checks have satisfied me that the experts know best. Once or twice I baulked e.g. at Pedretti's translation of "luce" by "cornea", but, on reflexion, I decided that, while not strictly correct, this rendering might make it easier for the non-specialist reader.

Now, I must confess to a sense of loss. Leonardo's was without question one of the great minds in depth and width. But it seems to me that his insight and ingenuity did not prevent him from making mistakes he could easily have avoided. The heights of greatness are lonely: perhaps he should have shared his ideas – much as Plato gives us to understand that he did – and, unlike Plato, he could have tested criticism by experiment, in the ingenuity of which he shone. But he did not, and that is that.

We must remember, however, that it is his ideas that he records, and that there are other records of what was going on at the time. He was a contemporary of the mad friar Girolamo Savonarola as he was of the Medici who had "made and undone" him. There had been the invasion of the French. And, even if Florence did not deal with him harshly as she had done once with Dante and, during Leonardo's life-time, with Michelangelo, he lived, a restless spirit, like most of humanity, in restless times. The occasional inconsistency in his reasoning, the odd non sequitur, are mere echoes perhaps of the breathlessness with which he was forced to do some of his work.

References

Dugaćki V. Prvi naš znanstventi traktat o fiziološkoj optici. (Our first known treatise on physiological optics). Jugosl oftalm arh 1977; 3: 4: 17–22.

Keele KD. Leonardo da Vinci's elements of the science of man. New York, London: Academic Press, 1983.

Documenta Ophthalmologica 68: 35–45 (1988)

Ophthalmological lore in the Corpus Hippocraticum

JOHN LASCARATOS & SPIROS MARKETOS

Department of History of Medicine, National University of Athens, Athens, Greece

Abstract. In this paper we examine the ophthalmological knowledge of the Hippocratic School as described in the Corpus Hippocraticum. An analysis is made of knowledge existing at the time concerning the anatomy of the eye and the physiology of vision, as well a diseases of the eye and ophthalmic surgical operations as depicted in the Corpus. In particular, the book "About Vision" from the Corpus Hippocraticum is discussed in detail. From our study of the extant texts it becomes apparent that not only was knowledge of ophthalmology considerably developed in the time of Hippocrates but it constituted a source of inspiration for ophthalmic treatments carried out by later physicians and in particular by those of the 19th century.

"If we wanted to confine ourselves to the authentic books by Hippocrates, we could cite only a few paragraphs on eye diseases. The School of Hippocrates had only little knowledge about ophthalmology. Unfortunately, we do not have a composite description of ophthalmology by the School of Hippocrates as we have it by the Indian ophthalmologists" [8]. This is how Hirschberg describes in his History of Ophthalmology the state of this branch of medical science in Hippocrates' day. Though Hirschberg's comment may be true of the authentic works of Hippocrates, we believe it lacks validity if we apply it to the complete works which make up the Corpus Hippocraticum, for, abundant examples may be found of the ophthalmological knowledge of the time which prove that the science was far from being disregarded by the Ancients. Besides, how could they neglect a branch which, according to the latest findings by Kavvadias and other archeologists, was highly developed at the ancient Asclepieia, where thousands of sufferers flocked to benefit from the ophthalmological services offered [17].

The Hippocratic School had a vague conception of the anatomy of the eye and it seems highly probable that dissections had been carried out on the eyes of animals. According to the information provided by the Corpus Hippocraticum, the eye is composed of "three sheaths, the outer-most being the thickest, the middle one slightly thinner, while the innermost, which contains the liquid, is the finest" (Littré, VI, 280).*

---

* Extracts from the ancient Greek have been translated from the original as it was felt that, where translations did exist, they did not do justice to the full meaning of the text. All numbers in the text refer to the edition of Littré [10].

Table 1.

1.	Various types of conjunctivitis
2.	Pterygium
3.	Sty
4.	Cellulitis
5.	Ectropion
6.	Diseases of the cilia
7.	Lacrymation with irritation of the eye
8.	Scabies
9.	Corneal Ulcers
10.	Epiphora
11.	Scars (four types) of the cornea
12.	Prolapse of the Iris
13.	Irregular pupil
14.	Dilated pupil
15.	Constricted pupil
16.	Change of colour of the pupil
17.	Amblyopia
18.	Amaurosis
19.	Hemianopia
20.	Dayblindness
21.	Floaters
22.	Photopsia
23.	Strabismus (concomitant and paralytic)
24.	Nystagmus (Hippus)
25.	Ulcerous Blepharitis

It also seems that the Hippocratic School was aware of the existence of the pupil, the iris, the vitreous and the crystal lens which are broadly described. There is evidence that the lacrymal system was also known, for the interconnection between nose and eye had been recognized though not clearly described. The eye is sustained by "veins, fine in appearance" which "pass from the brain through the surrounding sheath; these veins sustain vision by means of the purest liquid emanating from the brain" (VI, 278). Concerning the theory of vision, the Hippocratic School, in an attempt to reconcile conflicting earlier opinions, maintains that whether the eyes emit rays capable of producing the perception of objects, or whether the image is projected by the objects themselves, the phenomenon of vision is accomplished through movement. It is the vibration of the air, rather than radiation, which produces the phenomenon [12].

Vision is achieved by means of the extremely fine viscid substance from the brain which filters through the two veins connecting the brain to the eyes. Amblyopia is caused by the flow of phlegm from the brain through the veins of the eye and thus "vision becomes watery and blurred, the eye loses its luster and objects are not clearly visible" (VII, 8).

Moreover, concerning the perception of colour, we find in the Corpus Hippocraticum the remarkable observation that "Colours do not look the same at all times, nor when north or south winds blow, nor do they seem the same to all ages" (V, 500).

According to Hirschberg [8], a description of the following eye diseases and symptoms is to be found in the Corpus Hippocraticum (Table 1).

It is uncertain whether cataract is described in the Corpus Hippocraticum. Most probably the term "Glaucosis" referred to a clouding of the lens. The hypochyma which later physicians treated surgically is nowhere mentioned [18].

After Hippocrates, his successor Chrysippus makes first mention of the treatment of hypochyma by couching, so, however attractive, Professor Knapp's opinion that the overnight cure of patients at the Asklepieia, can be attributed to the probable depression of their hypochymas, seems to be baseless [1].

Other researchers [6, 7, 12] have discerned in the Hippocratic texts a perfect description of ophthalmic migraine (V, 444), the empirical measurement of visual acuity through the use of the fingers (VII, 284), trichiasis, trauma of the eyelids, lagophthalmos, blepharospasmus, Horner's syndrome, automatic regression of cataracts (V, 174), a clinical picture of vernal conjunctivitis and even a description of the Adamantiades-Behçet syndrome which, according to Feigenbaum, is to be found in Hippocrates' third book on epidemics, where the author mentions: "The mouths of many sufferers were aphthous and ulcerous. Their genitals were afflicted with defluxions and several ulcerations, persistent and painful . . . watery ophthalmias which caused blindness in many cases" [1].

Moreover, several researchers [2, 3, 4, 11, 15] have recognized the picture of trachoma from the descriptions given in the works of the Corpus Hippocraticum. Significant, too, is the observation of amaurosis of the eye following trauma to the eyebrow (V, 698), due, apparently, to injury to the optic nerve at its point of access through the optical canal. Mention is also made of the manifestation of ophthalmic symptoms in cases of cranial fracture (V, 624 and 696) and especially temporal fracture (V, 401).

Concerning surgical operations mentioned in the Corpus Hippocraticum, we know [5, 8, 11] of the following: (Table 2).

This last procedure of trephining the skull was carried out to relieve endocranial pressure in cases of amaurosis, due apparently to pressure on the optic nerve. Commenting on this point, Souques [12] writes: "These lines prove that the Hippocratic physicians were familiar with amaurosis due to oedema of the papilla i.e. to hypertension in the cerebrospinal fluid caused either by serous meningitis or a tumour of the brain".

Table 2.

1.	Scarification of granular conjunctiva
2.	The excision of thickened granular conjunctiva
3.	Draining of puss from the anterior chamber (hypopion)
4.	Surgical treatment of trichiasis
5.	Occasionally the removal of an arrowhead from the lid is mentioned
6.	Incisions into the skin of the head as well as cranial trephining are occasionally recommended for the treatment of eye diseases

"About Vision"

The book "Περί Οψιος" from the Corpus Hippocraticum is not, of course, one of Hippocrates' authentic works, of which, as we know, very few survived [16]. It has been suggested that the text was originally a part of the book "On suffering" or even that it was written by Polybus, Hippocrates' son-in-law. Other researchers have expressed the opinion that it belongs to the Alexandrine period [15]. Despite these rather far-fetched assertions the book is nowadays considered a part of the Corpus Hippocraticum.

The title indicates the contents of the book. In Hippocrates' day, the term "όψις" meant "vision", though at times it denoted the eye, the cornea, the iris and even, occasionally, the pupil [15]. The title has been translated to "About Vision" and this interpretation prevails in foreign language translations. Only the famous ophthalmologist and historian, Kostomires, maintained that the title should be translated as "About the Eye" [14]. The book has survived in a mutilated state. Unquestionably, large excerpts are missing from the text, thus making it impossible for us to arrive at a clear conclusion regarding the level attained by ophthalmology of those times, though the few fragments that remain indicate that the Hippocratic School's knowledge of the subjects must have been considerable [11].

A total of nine chapters have survived. The first chapter of "About Vision" concerns changes in the colour of the eyes and various diseases. "Damaged eyes", we are told, "automatically acquire a deep blue colour, and once this has happened there is no cure. When eyes take on the colour of the sea they gradually deteriorate over a long period of time or one eye is destroyed while the other gradually follows" [9, 11]. Certain researchers have recognized in this picture a description of glaucoma [12, 18].

The second chapter refers to disturbances of vision without any change in the colour of the eyes. The writer recommends that when young people with impaired vision reach full development, the thickness of their eyelids should be reduced by means of scraping and mild cauterization.

The third chapter is the most important, for it gives the necessary instructions for cauterizing veins and, in general, for all cauterization, which seems to have been a major therapeutic procedure of the times. Cauterizations were performed preferably over the backbone. After an outline of the veins had been traced on the skin, cauterization would be carried out with thick iron instruments in gradual stages so that haemorhaging would not occur during the treatment. Then a sponge soaked in oil would be placed upon the cauterized spot in such a way as to deepen the burn, while avoiding the proximity of the bone. After this, the sores were covered with a concoction of honey and Dracunculus vulgaris.

The fourth chapter of the book concerns the scraping and cauterization of granulomas of the lid. In the treatment for this disease, Greek ophthalmologists of the past, such as Anagnostakis, have also discerned a therapeutic method for trachomas. It was on this extract from the Corpus Hippocraticum that the estimable Woolhouse based his claim to be the first to discover the importance of the work which had previously been unappreciated by Greeks and Latins alike. Though most people know the story of Woolhouse, whom Sichel considered a charlatan, they are unaware of the existence of Woolhouse's Greek counterpart.

This was George Kostomires, an ophthalmologist and otologist from Mytilene (Lesbos) who, at the meeting of the Greek Medical Association of 13th November, 1882, presented a new method for the treatment of trachomas [7]. Kostomires' announcement was immediately challenged by his fellow ophthalmologists, Prof. Anagnostakis among them, who doubted the efficacy of his treatment and claimed it was a Hippocratic method. Kostomires' treatment consisted of rubbing the trachomatic conjunctivas with a concoction made up of water, glycerine ointment, white mercury precipitate, boric acid and wild basil [7]. It does seem, however, that Kostomires had been inspired by the Hippocratic texts, for he was well-versed in Ancient Greek, an ardent admirer of the Ancients and a serious scholar of ancient texts. Even his thesis, published in 1893 in Paris, dealt with apobrochism, which was a Hippocratic treatment for trichiasis [14]. He had already concerned himself with this method previously and had submitted a treatise on "The treatment of trichiasis by hypotomy followed by resuturing" at the Greek Medical Association's meeting of 10th November, 1879. Moreover, Kostomires had advocated licking as a therapeutic method for corneal ulcers, inspired no doubt by the treatment provided at the ancient Asklepieia, where the licking of ulcers by snakes and dogs was practised [17]. The opprobrium that Kostomires' opinions brought upon him was no less than that suffered by Woolhouse in his time.

The relevant Hippocratic text dealing with the treatment of granulomas of the lid reads thus: "When the eye-lid has to be scraped, do this first and then cauterize it with a shuttle-shaped piece of wood, wrapped in clean, curly wool from Miletus, taking care all the while to avoid the corona* of the eye and not to allow the cauter to reach the cartilage. The sign that cauterization should proceed no deeper is when the flow of bright blood ceases and is replaced by ichor.** After this some liquid medicament containing copper "bloom" should be applied to the lids" [9, 11].

Anagnostakis considered the above to be the earliest significant treatment of trachoma, and the subject was interminably discussed with Sichel who published his well-known treatise in Littré though Anagnostakis considered that the translation at several points left much to be desired. This scientific controversy was finally concluded with Sichel's acceptance of many of Anagnostakis' views [2, 3, 4, 5, 19, 20, 21]. Anagnostakis believed that this method, which derives from the Corpus Hippocraticum, had been perpetuated by general practicians in the Greek countryside up to his time. Of course, the therapeutic qualities of copper in the treatment of trachomas are well-known to this day.

The fifth chapter of the Corpus deals with fleshy granulomas and recommends that when the lids are thicker than normal they should be cut away from beneath and then mildly cauterized. According to this text, over-development of the lid can be prevented by the application of burnt copper bloom [9, 11].

The sixth chapter concerns erosive catarrhal ophthalmia. When the lids are eroded and itching occurs, it states, we crush a small piece of copper bloom on a whetting stone and then rub it onto the lid. The text goes on to give further instructions on the use of various concoctions for the treatment of the disease [8, 9, 11].

The seventh chapter is also of particular significance, for it concerns the treatment of nyctalopia. It recommends that patients suffering from this disease should be given the juice of the wild cucumber as well as ox-liver soaked in honey. Dry cupping should be carried out over the back of the neck [9, 11]. Of all these therapeutic treatments, the most rational, which was in fact adhered to throughout the following ages and is mentioned by many great physicians of later times, is the use of ox-liver whose therapeutic efficacy is attributed to the abundance of Vitamin A it contains. However, it is apparent from the Hippocratic text that the term nyctalopia did not

* It is not known what exactly Hippocrates meant by this term. Some historians believe he meant the limbus, others that the "corona" indicated the cornea, and Anagnostakis himself took the term to mean the edge of the lids [2, 3, 4, 5].
** In the 19th century "ichor" was taken to refer to a purulent, malodorous greenish liquid, exuded by wounds. In Homeric epics, however, "ichor" referred to the liquid circulating in the veins of the gods. In this text it has the meaning of "a serous secretion, containing traces of blood".

signify as it does today impairment of vision at night, but rather diminished vision in daytime, and this is why Anagnostakis makes the tentative suggestion that the term might have signified simple photophobia – although this does not correspond with the treatment with raw ox-liver [2, 3].

The eighth chapter, which is also of particular interest, refers to the treatment of amaurosis by trephining the cranium. "Should a person with healthy eyes be afflicted with loss of vision, the skin over the bregmatic region should be cut away, the cranial bone beneath sawed into, and when the collected liquid is removed the patient is cured" [9, 11]. This is the well-known extract discussed by Souques, as we mention above [12].

The ninth chapter which refers to epidemic conjunctivitis recommends thorough cleansing of the head and lower abdomen and, if the patient's constitution permits, bleeding. The patient is recommended a diet of bread, in small quantity, and water. His bed should be in a dark place, far from smoke, fire and any bright object, and he should lie on his side [9, 11]. The instruction that the patient should lie in a darkened room is significant as this would of course avoid photophobia, while smoke and fire would certainly aggravate his condition. The text goes on to give the following directions [9, 11]: "The patient should avoid looking at anything intensely or steadily, as this causes watering of the eyes, for the eye cannot bear to gaze on anything bright.On the other hand, nor must he allow his eyes to remain closed for any length of time, especially when there is a flow of hot tears, for tears confined to the eye heat and irritate it".

From all the above it is apparent that if the book "About Vision" had survived in its entirety, we would have a far better picture of Hippocratic ophthalmology and many points in the texts would have become clear.

Furthermore, even in its extant mutilated state, the work can in no way be considered insignificant, seeing that certain extracts have inspired therapeutic methods on a Greek and even on an international scale, while others have given rise to numerous controversies and certainly a great deal of speculation. We have mentioned Woolhouse's therapeutic treatment, Kostomires' surgical and pharmaceutic methods and the opinions of Anagnostakis, who maintained that the Hippocratic text provides the earliest description of trachoma and the first reference to treatment with "wool from Melitos" wrapped round a wooden shuttle, the very same method on which Woolhouse based the therapy that made him famous [2, 3, 4, 5, 19, 20, 21]. At the same time, certain therapeutic treatments, such as that for nyctalopia, seem quite reasonable today. Even the treatment for amaurosis by trephining the skull seems, in the light of present knowledge, perfectly rational, though it must have been inexplicable in the past. Some of the references to the treatment of conjunctivities, later supplemented by Alexander Trallionos, are remarkable and could reasonably be employed today in the prevailing conditions of atmospheric pollution.

We hope that the evidence we presented above illuminates the Hippocratic School's considerable contribution to the development of ophthalmology and its influence on the thinking of ophthalmologists many centuries later. The most remarkable point, however, is that the Hippocratic School perceived ophthalmic diseases and symptoms in a broader functional context. Far from being isolated or considered local manifestations, they were seen as an expression of the complete nosological entity. From the "Fixed stare" (Κατάπληξη ομμάτων) and the "Glaring Squint" (Θράσος ομμάτων ιλλωδέων) both symptoms of more general cerebral disturbance, to Polymedes or Farsala's reference to oedema of the lids (considered by Sichel as a possible expression of Bright's disease) everything points unquestionably to the affinity between ophthalmology and every disease man is prone to. Centuries later in Paris, another enlightened ophthalmologist, Professor Fotinos Panas, arrived at the same conclusion, for he would advise his pupils not to limit their studies to ophthalmology pure and simple, but to acquire a complete and more comprehensive knowledge of medicine if they wished to do justice to their vocation.

Apart, however, from its purely scientific contribution, a work which dealt with all branches of medicine could not disregard matters of professional conduct. So, on the principle that "Υγιέας ποιείν πάντας αδύνατον" ("It is impossible to heal everyone"), Hippocrates consoles doctors when their best efforts result in failure. "When we treat the eyes and anoint them, the pain may worsen, the eyes may rupture and become blind. Then the doctor is blamed and accused of being neglectful". (VI, 154).

In a time like the present, when dominant and influential ophthalmological opinions are overturned in short order and rendered obsolete by the ineluctable march of scientific progress, the Hippocratic insistence on holistic treatment of ophthalmic disorders seems particularly relevant to modern thinking.

References

1. Adams F. The Genuine works of Hippocrates. Vol I. London: Syndenham Society. 1849; 399–403.
2. Anagnostakis A. Concerning the Hippocratic method of scraping and cauterizing trachomatic lids. A comment on Sichel's interpretation. Medical Journal (Athens) 1860; 73: 177–183.
3. Anagnostakis A. Della Baschiatura e della cauterizzazione delle palpebre granellose secondo Ippocrate. Giornale d'Oftalmologia Italiano 1860; 3: 11.

4. Anagnostakis A. Contributions historiques à la pathologie et à la therapeutique des granulations palpebrales. Extrait du Comte-Rendu du Congrès d'Ophtalmologie de Paris 1862; 40–55.

5. Anagnostakis A. Contributions à l'histoire de la chirurgie oculaire chez les anciens. Ann D'Ocul 1870; 63: 97–107.

6. Feigenbaum A. Description of Behçet's syndrome in the Hippocratic Third Book of Endemic Diseases. Brit J Ophthal 1956; 40: 355–357.

7. Gabrielides K. Ophthalmology during the course of the existence of the Medical Association 1835–1932. Bulletin of the Medical Association of Athens 1933; 501–523.

8. Hirschberg J. The History of Ophthalmology, Vol I. Transl Blodi F. Bonn: JP Wayenborgh, 1982; 59–134.

9. Hippocrates. Omnia Opera Hippocratis. Aldus, Venetiis. 1526. Hippocrates "About Vision", p. 224.

10. Hippocrates. Omnia Opera. Paris: E. Littré, 1839–1861.

11. Hippocrates. Complete works. Vol. E. About Vision. Preface by G. Pournaropoulos. Translated into modern Greek by K. Emmanuel. Athens: Edition Martinis SA, pp. 526–541.

12. Kastrandas AD. Ophthalmological knowledge of the Ancient Greeks in the time of Hippocrates. Athens, 1960.

13. Knapp P. Zur Frage der Staroparation bei den alten Griechen. Klin Mbl Augenheilk 1930; 84: 277–279.

14. Kostomires GA. Recherches et commentaires sur l'apobronchisme. Operation hippocratique du trichiasis etc. Thèses, Paris. Arch D'Ophtal 1893; 13: 641.

15. Kostomires GA. Concerning Ophthalmology and Otology in Ancient Greece from the earliest times to Hippocrates' day. Athens, 1887.

16. Kouzes AP. The History of Medicine Athens, 1929.

17. Lascaratos J. Ophthalmological treatment in the Asclepeia. Greek Annals of Ophthalmology 1980; 17: 143–154.

18. Lascaratos J, Marketos S. The cataract operation in Ancient Greece. Histoire des Sciences Médicales 1982; 17: 317–322.

19. Sichel J. Hippocrate de la vision. Paris: JB Baillière et fils, 1860.

20. Sichel J. Note complémentaire sur le traitement chirurgical des granulations palpébrales exposé dans un des livres Hippocratiques. Ann D'Ocul 1861; 65.

21. Sichel J. Note complémentaire sur le traité de la vision d'Hippocrate. Paris: JB Baillière et fils, 1861.

Address for offprints: John Lascaratos, M.D.,9, Or. Taxiarchias Str. Zografou, Athens 1572, Greece

Glossary of ophthalmological terms in ancient Greek texts

Achyls: Superficial, extensive or complete ulceration of the cornea, leading to leucoma.

Aegylops: purulent dacryocystitis, which has ruptured, and fistulated.

Anchylops: purulent dacryocystitis. (In ancient texts this refers to an

	inflamed collection of pus between the internal canthus and the nose).
Apostema:	a collection of pus, frequently inflamed. In ancient texts this refers to sties.
Argemon:	small ulcer of the limbus.
Bothrion:	small, circular, clean ulcer of the cornea.
Coeloma:	ulcer similar to, but wider than, the bothrion.
Eganthis:	fleshy outgrowth near the internal canthus, probably a fleshy caruncle.
Eccauma:	scabby ulcer of the cornea.
Epicauma:	grey-coloured, rough textured, putrid ulcer of the cornea leading to possible rupture.
Helon:	an advanced form of staphyloma, associated with total blindness. Ancient Greek medical writers graded staphylomas (which they named proptoses) on a scale of severity. The least severe was myocephalon, followed by staphyloma (meaning "grape-sized"), melon (where the choroid protrudes beyond the eyelid) and helon.
Hypochyma:	supposed pathological liquid secretion, between the cornea and the lens, which was transformed into a membrane. When ancient doctors removed, or "couched" cataracts, they believed they were removing this imaginary membrane. In the 19th century this term described cataracts in general.
Milphosis:	Madarosis. In ancient texts this term was associated with the modern alopecia.
Myocephalon:	small staphyloma, the size of fly's head. (mya = fly, cephale = head).
Nephelion:	superficial scar of the cornea, also called Ouli (= scar). When this extends to the inner layers of the cornea it becomes a leucoma. Some ancient writers use this term to describe a small, deep ulcer of the cornea, causing slight opaqueness.
Paremptosis:	total blindness caused by obstruction of the optic "spirit" (according to the well-known ancient theories on vision).
Psorophthalmia:	a form of blepharitis combined with conjunctivitis, causing tears, ulceration of the canthi, inflamation and itching of the eyelids.
Ptilosis:	madarosis, combined with xerophthalmia and thickening of the rims of the eyelids.
Rhyas:	a condition in which tears, instead of flowing normally

through the tear duct, overflow the eye at the internal canthus.

Sycosis: a form of trachoma. According to the ancients, "trachoma" described a roughness of the inner eyelid. When the roughness was severe and the conjunctiva of the lids was chapped, the condition ws called Sycosis. When the same condition became chronic and hard lumps appeared on the conjunctiva, it was called "Tylosis".

Taraxis: mild conjunctivitis.

Tyle: Tylosis. (See Sycosis).

Documenta Ophthalmologica 68: 47–56 (1988)
© Kluwer Academic Publishers, Dordrecht

The representation of the eye in African and Oceanian art

PIERRE AMALRIC

Albi, France

Everyday, it is proven that Africa has been the cradle of human race. The first traces of man and, consequently of his culture, are located in Olduvai Gorges, to the East of Lake Victoria, in Tanzania.

If we refer to the XVth and XVIth century cartography initiated by the Arabs or the Portuguese, we are immediately struck by the isolation and the lack of knowledge of Europeans concerning African life (Fig. 1).

However, we know that, as early as this period, the works of art which were brought back to Europe could easily be integrated into the collections of Roman Catholic Kings.

Several periods are important in the evolution of the knowledge of African Art:

— 1486: The Portuguese Diago Cao gives several African works of art to Charles the Bold.

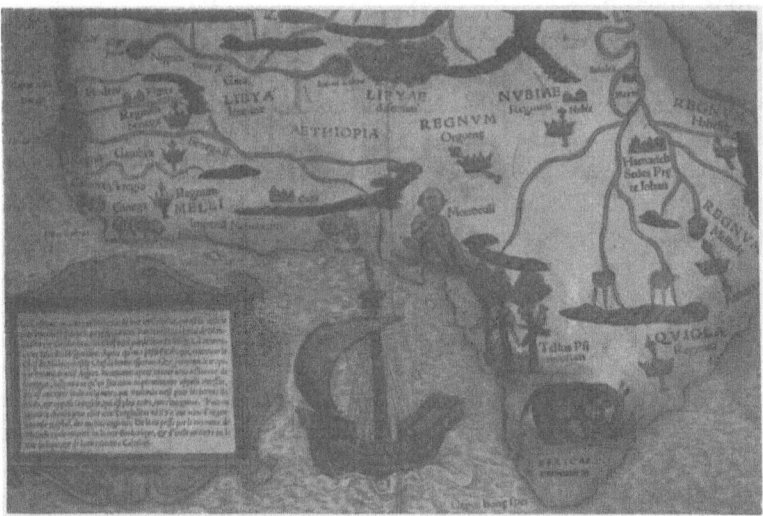

Fig. 1. Map of Africa. XVIth century (private collection).

— 1527: Francis I receives several African works of art from Dieppe sailors.
— XVIIth century: in Rome, Kircher, a Jesuit, founds the first African Museum with several statues from the Congo.
— 1668: Dapper (Holland) describes the capital of Benin.

By the end of the XIXth century, the German ethnologue, Leo Frobenius, undertook the first major survey of Africanism. Two Englishmen, Read and Dalton, discover the Benin Art and in France, the Trocadéro Ethnographic Museum is unaugurated in 1879.

Important exhibitions were dedicated to Africa, in Leipzig (1892), in Antwerp (1894) and before the opening of the Belgian Congo Museum at Brussels-Tervuren in 1897.

By the beginning of the XXth century, three major books on African art were published in Europe. Henri Clouzot and André Level edited the first French book on the subject: *L'Art Nègre et l'Art Océanien,* Paris, Ed. Devambez, 1919; in Germany, Leo Frobenius published *Das Unbekannte Afrika*, München, C. Beck'sche Verlag, 1923 and in England, Robert Sutherland Rattray published *Ashanti*, Oxford, Clarendon Press, 1923.

The beginning of the XXth century corresponds to the great period of initiation in African and Oceanian art.

Some painters such as Picasso and Maurice de Vlaminck realized the interest that this art might present for some European artists in search of new techniques. The latter considered Negro art in all its primitivism and in all its grandeur.

In 1906–1907, Picasso painted "Les Demoiselles d'Avignon" where, on the right side of the painting, the form was created by parallel lines of colour, which announce cubism. With this work, Picasso inaugurated his "negro period", characterized by figures whose sharply marked features evoked those of African sculptures.

Other painters, such as Derain who originated fauvism, Marcel Duchamp who promoted the Dadaist movement together with Picabia who made a painting called "Chanson Nègre" in 1913, underwent the same influence.

In sculpture, the cubist school was also inspired by African Art.

Guillaume Apollinaire wrote in 1912 a poem entitled "Zone" where the Negro African theme appears for the first time.

In Germany, an exhibition on Black Art was presented at the Folkwangmuseum in Hagen in 1912 and Carl Einstein published *Negerplastik* (Leipzig, Verlag der Weissen Bücher, 1915) where the major qualities of African sculptures are outlined.

In Zürich, Tristan Tzara, one of the founders of the Dadaist movement, observed in his article (published in Paris in the journal "Sic") that "Sym-

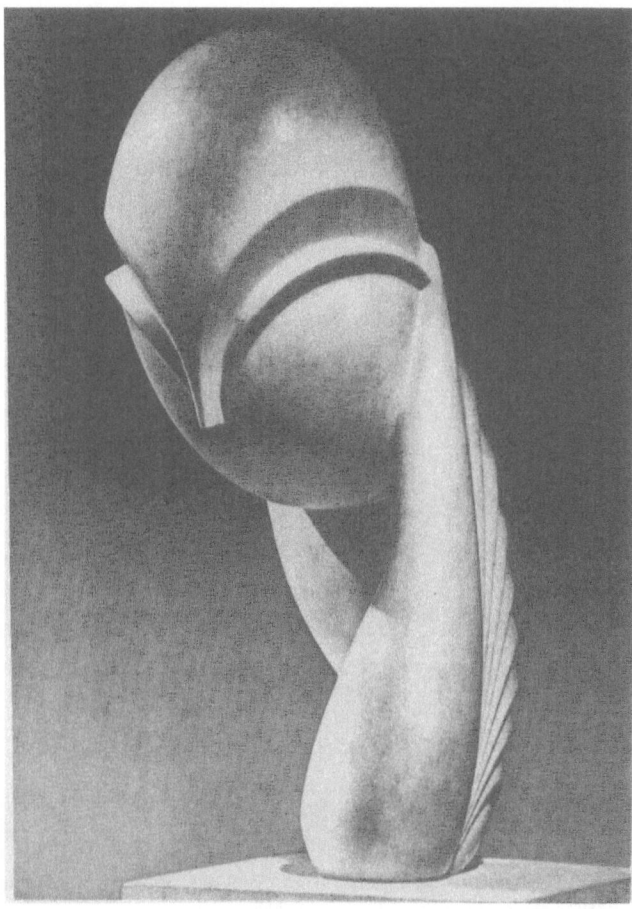

Fig. 2a. Constantin Brancusi. Miss Pogany, 1931. In: Duchamp et son temps. Ed. Time Life. Le monde des arts. Time Life International, 1973, p. 45.

metry and verticality are very important to the African painter. He concentrates his vision on the head and loses the conventional proportion of head to body".

Since the beginning of the century, the concordances and similarities between African and Modern Art have become increasingly obvious. (Figs. 2a and 2b).

If some artists, as Picasso, deny this evidence, others acknowledge it. On comparing Klee, Lipchitz, Santini, Modigliani and Brancusi's works with African or Oceanian masks, we can find a common inspiration. The discovery of vases made in remote Antiquity in Jericho 3.000 years B.C. or in the

50

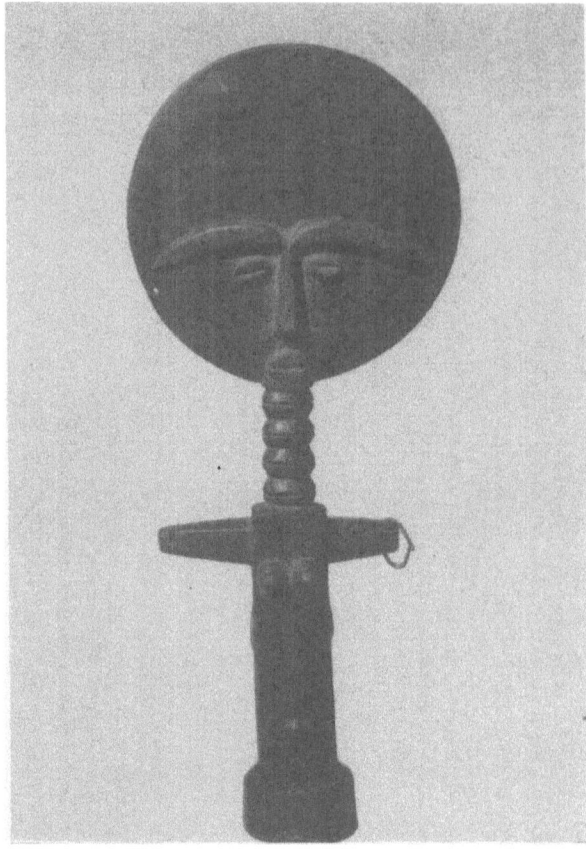

Fig. 2b. Statue from Guinea (private collection). In: Michel Leiris and Jacqueline Delonge. Afrique noire. Paris: Gallimard, 1967, Fig. 113, p. 118.

Middle-East during the same period, reveal the same inspiration. The eye is magnified in relation to the face and this symbolism is increased by symmetry. Either on top of a stick or on a stone, the eye occupies a privileged position in the face of Hittite gods.

The symbol of the eye, characteristic of human beings, is very rarely neglected in African Art. Moreover, apart from rare exceptions, the axis of the head and body is always vertical.

As far as we are concerned, we are struck by the persistence of some characteristics: the head is almost always the essential element of the work. The sculptor creates a disproportion between the head which he magnifies and the body which he reduces.

In African Art, the representation of the head goes from the most complete anatomical objectivity to the most excessive surrealism. However, one of the essential elements is the concern for symmetry with the median line. The eyes are situated on both sides of the ridge of the nose which is always considered as the main axis for the composition of the whole work.

It seems extremely rare to find eyes represented in the middle of the face. Sometimes, they may correspond to only two orifices marked in the wood or the metal; often, their size is normal but more usually it is considerably magnified.

Diverse influences can be defined in African Art, according to three main areas of the continent. The first one, located around the Sénégal and Niger Rivers, gave rise to Nok Art. The second area, corresponding to the Guinea

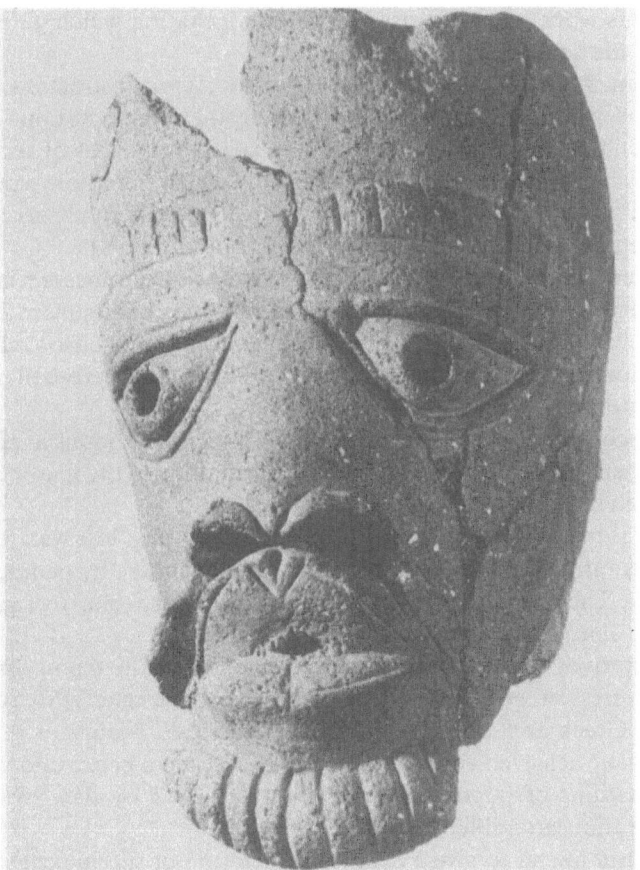

Fig. 3. Nok statute with triangular-shaped eyes. Vth century B.C. In: Mary Cable. Les chefs Africains. Ed. Time Life. Coll. Les trésors de l'histoire. Cop. Ed. du Fanal, 1984, p. 14.

coast from Cape Coast to Cameroun, covered important centers in Nigeria and Ghana which embraced the life, Benin, Edo and Ibo civilizations. The third area is located in Congo, from Gabon to Angola and North Rhodesia, and it included numerous civilizations, among others the Bakouba and the Bakongo civilizations.

Sculptures produced by these diverse civilizations are extremely variable in their conception. However, they present some constant characteristics. The African artist intended first of all to emphasize the religious factor in the choice of his subjects. He meant to express the importance of the family and the cult of ancestors.

Wood was the most commonly used material, which explains the non-preservation of most ancient works of African sculptures, though, to preserve his work, the artist used a protective coating which gave a special patina to the sculpture.

In Sudan, Mali or Senegal, the art expresses a lyric abstraction with great intensity in its anthropomorphic or zoomorphic representation.

The rectangular-shaped eye is symmetrical on both sides of the nose and appears as being the essential element around which the whole work is built. These sculptures, which are most appreciated by modern artists, date back to very remote times with regard to their inspiration.

However, the first artistic manifestations have been located in Nigeria, according to actual researches. In Nok, terra-cottas dating from 2 centuries B.C. have been discovered. Their original conception is based on a similar presentation of the eye: triangular palpebral slip, tubular eye-ball perforated in the center, well drawn eyebrow-arch. (Fig. 3).

The discovery of Benin Art in the XIXth century posed a problem to archeologists. Since then, we have got confirmation of the filiation between the Nok civilization and modern sculptures.

Bronze is much used in Benin Art, according to the "lost wax technique" which was introduced at the end of the XIIIth century by people from Ifé in Nigeria. The characteristics of portraiture are particularly original in Ifé art with a sharp naturalistic tendency.

The purity of forms, the precision of details and the dignity of attitude give an impression of majestuous serenity which characterize Ifé sculptures, recall the Greek archaic style and evoke "classical" beauty.

The artistic achievements of this period enable us to better understand the transformations of human representation achieved by the African artist through a thousand different aspects.

We do not intend to give a detailed description of specific characteristics corresponding to every region or tribe.

Some sculptures give the impression of being real aristocratic effigies.

Eyebrows are differently drawn, depending on whether the eyes are opened or closed.

Africa is the land of masks and, though all the peoples of the world have designed masks, their diversity and quantity is unique on this continent.

The originality of the artist is expressed in different types of masks. The modelling is completed by the patina and often by white painting.

The attitude of the face, with half-closed eyes, is meant to evoke death in silence and recollection, or seems to seek a privileged relation with death.

In some other cases, the predominance of eye-balls is maintained, in spite of stylization. The eyebrows are strongly marked and their arch, which joins

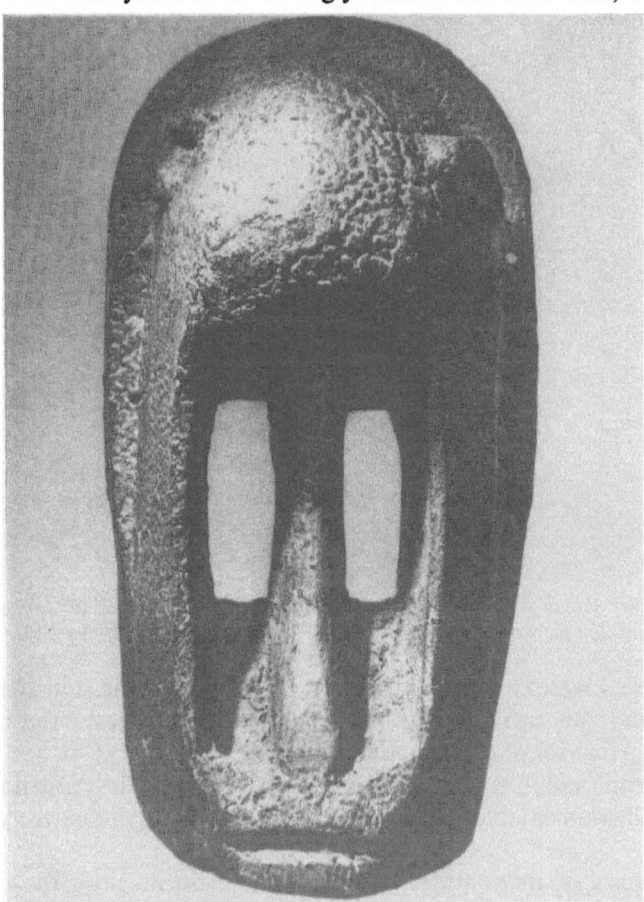

Fig. 4. Dogon art. Black Monkey, mask. Paris, Musée de l'Homme. In: Michel Leiris et Jacqueline Delonge. Afrique noire, la création artistique. Paris: Gallimard, 1967, Fig. 304, p. 270.

54

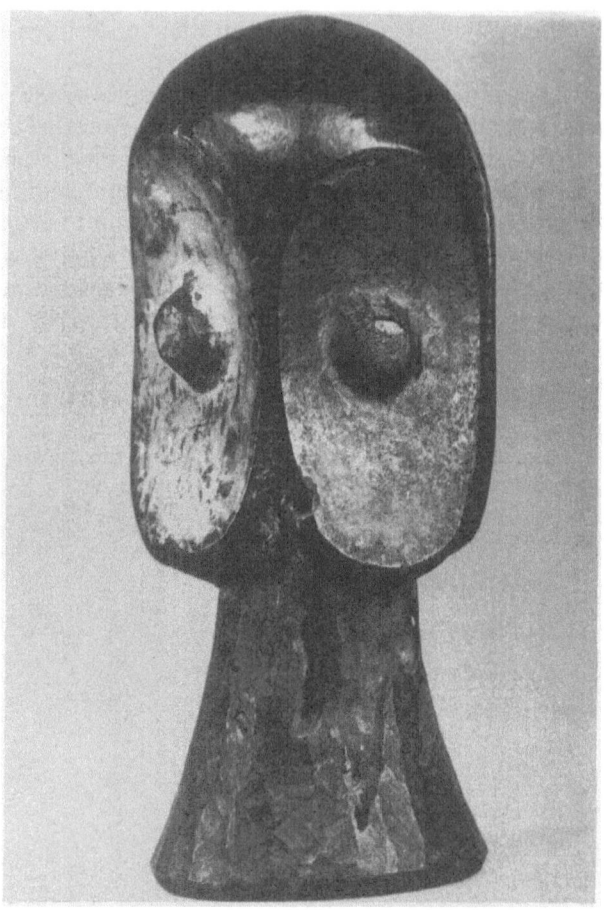

Fig. 5. Bembe art. Kalunga statute. Coll. René Vander Straete, Bruxelles. In: J. Cornet. Art de l'Afrique noire au pays du fleuve Zaire. Bruxelles: Ed. Arcade, 1972, Fig. 119, p. 228.

over the nose, creates another separation between the head and the eyes.

Tattoes and concentric radial lines which are painted over the face increase the surrealism of the representation.

The African sculptor may sometimes go beyond this evocation and achieve a schematization of the face showing only two symmetric eyeballs. (Figs. 4, 5).

In other cases, on the contrary, added tubular elements bring the eye into relief.

The sculptor may also represent a regular and complex striation around the eyes and cheeks, as it is the case in some tribes. These lines, running from the median axis around the eyes and mouth, enable the artist to outline both eyeballs.

The most essential element in African Art is the permanent care of all African artists to represent symmetric eyes on both sides of the nose, which differentiates them from Western artists who often break this harmony.

To conclude this short evocation consecrated to African Art, we shall quote the thought of two artists belonging to the Cubist School, who contributed to an important article entitled "Opinions sur l'Art Nègre".

"Les sculptures nègres nous donnent une preuve flagrante de la possibilité d'un art anti-idealiste. Animées de l'esprit religieux, elles sont des manifestations diverses et precises de grands principes et d'idées générales. Comment peut-on ne pas admettre un art qui procédant de cette façon arrive à individualiser ce qui est général et chaque fois d'une façon différente? Il est le contraire de l'art grec qui se basait sur l'individu pour essayer de suggérer un type idéal".

(Juan Gris. In: Action. Opinions sur l'Art Nègre. Paris, 1920; 23–26.

"L'art des nègres nous fut un grand exemple: leur vraie compréhension de la proportion, leur sentiment du dessin, leurs sens aigu de la réalité, nous ont fait entrevoir, oser même, beaucoup de choses".

(Jacques Lipchitz. In: Action. Opinions sur l'Art Nègre. Paris, 1920; 23–26.

Translations

"African sculpture, imbued with a religious spirit, embodies general ideas in many different, *individual* works of art. It is the very opposite of (classical) Greek art which based itself on the individual human in order to suggest an ideal type".

Juan Gris (In: Action. Opinions sur l'Art Nègre. Paris, 1920; 23–26. Editor's translation)

"African art served as a great example: their real understanding of proportion, their feeling for the drawing, their acute sense of reality have brought us to perceive, even to dare, many things".
Jacques Lipchitz. (In: Opinions sur l'Art Nègre. Paris, 1920; 23–26. Author's translation)

Oceanian Art is related to African Art in many respects.

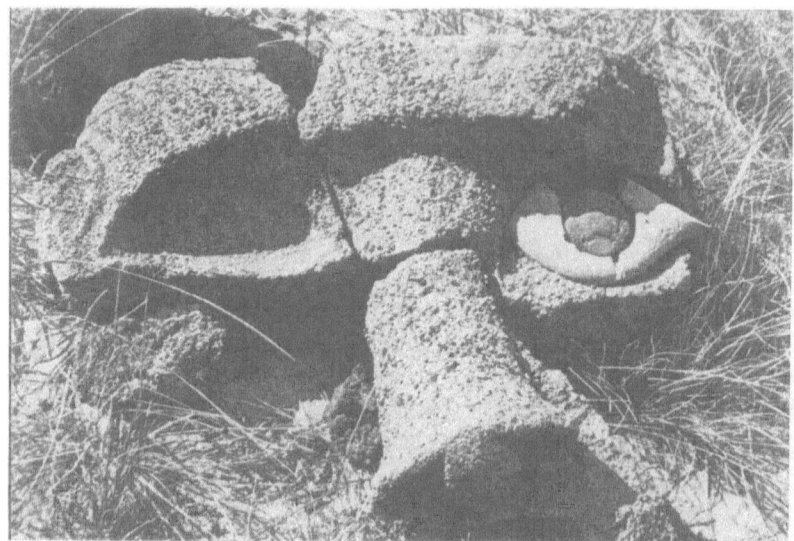

Fig. 6. Easter Island statute with its eye which was reconstituted. In: Rafa Nui. Nouveau regard sur l'Ile de Pâques. Cop. Moana Ed., 1982, p. 34.

The difference lies in an extraordinary polymorphism of colours and forms.

Using fragile materials, the Oceanian artist also lets the face prevail in his work: concentric circles, close relation between man and nature, use of corals, which result in a riot of modes representing the eye.

The spiral reveals dynamism and is observed in Maori tribes, as it was the case in Inca art.

The eye, which establishes this contact with life, is schematized by a spiral.

Being also a weapon, the eye is designed, with its size and gleam, to create terror on masks.

On the Easter Islands, the recent discoveries of the eyes of the statues (Fig. 6) show that the eye is the major element in the life of human beings and that it is necessary for their equilibrium.

Documenta Ophthalmologica 68: 57–63 (1988)

The Utrecht Ophthalmic Hospital and the development of tonometry in the 19th century

ISOLDE DEN TONKELAAR,[1] HAROLD E. HENKES[2] & GIJSBERT K. VAN LEERSUM[1]
[1] Royal Netherlands Ophthalmic Hospital, Utrecht; [2] Department of Ophthalmology, Erasmus University Rotterdam, the Netherlands

Abstract. During the second half of the 19th century Donders, Snellen and co-workers of the Utrecht Eye Clinic played an important role in the development of clinical tonometry. These indefatigable researchers designed and built a number of tonometers of which most have been saved and which are now on display in a permanent exhibition in the Royal Netherlands Ophthalmic Hospital at Utrecht.

The need for a more accurate measurement of intra-ocular pressure became apparent when Albrecht von Graefe reported in 1857 his successful treatment of acute glaucoma by means of an iridectomy.

In 1862, von Graefe himself designed the first ophthalmotonometer (Fig. 1), which was, however, not published. In a paper which appeared several years later Monnik, a trainee of Donders (see below) described von Graefe's tonometer but he did not give an illustration of the apparatus. Most probably the only still extant specimen is in the collection of the Utrecht Eye Clinic.

Von Graefe tried to determine the depth of the indentation after applying a given force to the sclera. However, in order to be able to use the instrument, the patient had to be examined under general anaesthesia (chloroform).

Another serious drawback was the point of reference given by the frontal bone and the upper jaw bone, as during the measurement the plunger not only indented the sclera but also pushed the eye into the orbit. In short, this instrument was certainly inadequate. Most likely, it was never used in the clinic.

Unaware of the fact that a specimen of A. von Graefe's tonometer was kept in the Utrecht clinic, Draeger (1961) had a reconstruction made based upon the description published by Monnik. However, he presumed that it had to be placed on the closed eyelid although Monnik had stated that the instrument was designed to be used on the sclera.

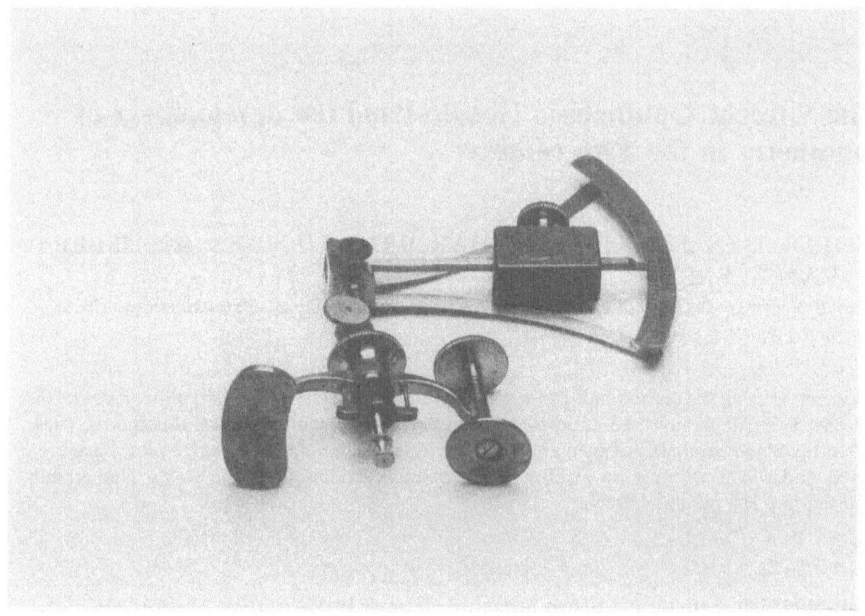

Fig. 1. Ophthalmotonometer of A. von Graefe (1862).

Almost simultaneously with but independently of von Graefe, Hamer, a trainee of Donders (who suggested its construction: Donders 1863) designed a tonometer of which only the interior parts have been preserved (Fig. 2, left). The rod which indented the sclera was connected with a pointer via a small toothed bar and wheelwork. However, this instrument also was not successful because the bar had to overcome too much friction resistance which made the measurements unreliable.

In another attempt Hamer tried to reduce the friction by inserting tiny copper bars along which the toothed bar moved. However, again friction problems emerged so that the instrument could not function properly. Moreover, its use required too much cooperation of the patient, let alone a highly skilled examiner. Hamer's second model (Fig. 2, center) still exists in its original form in the Utrecht instrument collection.

However, Donders, Hamer's mentor, did not give up. He requested a third model to be constructed (Fig. 2, right), in which the wheelwork was replaced by small levers. Yet this instrument suffered from the same imperfections as the former ones (Monnik, 1868).

Draeger was convinced that this instrument was the first model of Donders/Hamer, but the detailed description of Monnik clearly showed that it was in fact the third model.

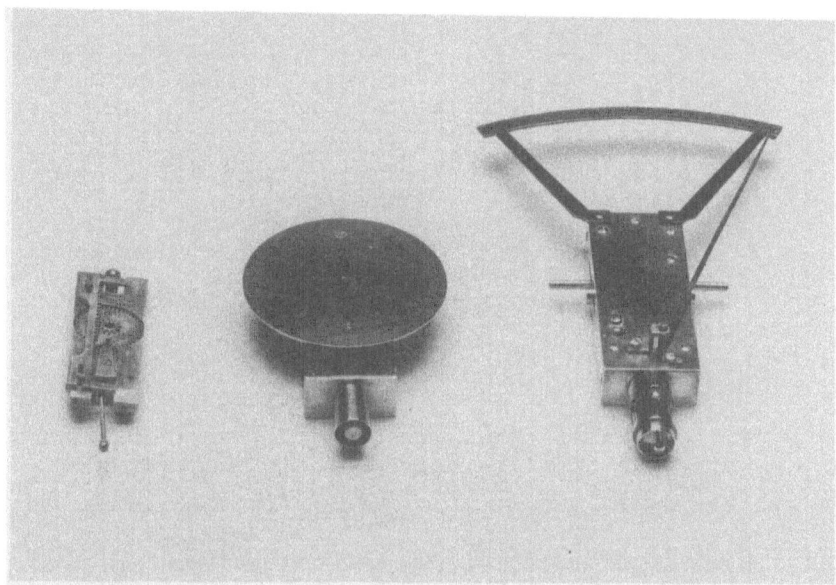

Fig. 2. (Left) tonometer of Hamer/Donders (1863). Only the interior parts have been preserved; (center) second model of Hamer/Donders; (right) third model, also constructed in 1863. From the outside it bears great similarity to the Schiøtz tonometer of 1905, but the construction is essentially different.

Still Donders refused to give in. He turned to Dor in Bern for help. Dor had received part of his training (like many of the prominent ophthalmologists of the second half of the 19th century) at the Utrecht Eye Clinic. Donders asked him to find a good watch-maker in Switzerland who seemed to be capable to construct a reliable tonometer. Dor commissioned Lecoultre, a famous watch-maker in Geneva to carry out the work. The resulting instrument was demonstrated by Dor at the 1865 – Heidelberg meeting, the year in which the design was published. Unfortunately, it also fell short of the expectations, one reason being again that too much friction resulted in unreliable results.

Meanwhile Donders did not just wait for the Swiss tonometer to be constructed, but wrote to Wheatstone in London (known from the Wheatstone's bridge). He asked him whether he could recommend someone capable to construct an instrument with the least possible friction resistance. Wheatstone recommended his own instrumentmaker, Mr. Stroh. Stroh indeed, succeeded in constructing a tonometer with very little friction (Fig. 3, left), but the instrument was too difficult to operate for being useful in daily practice (Monnik, 1868).

60

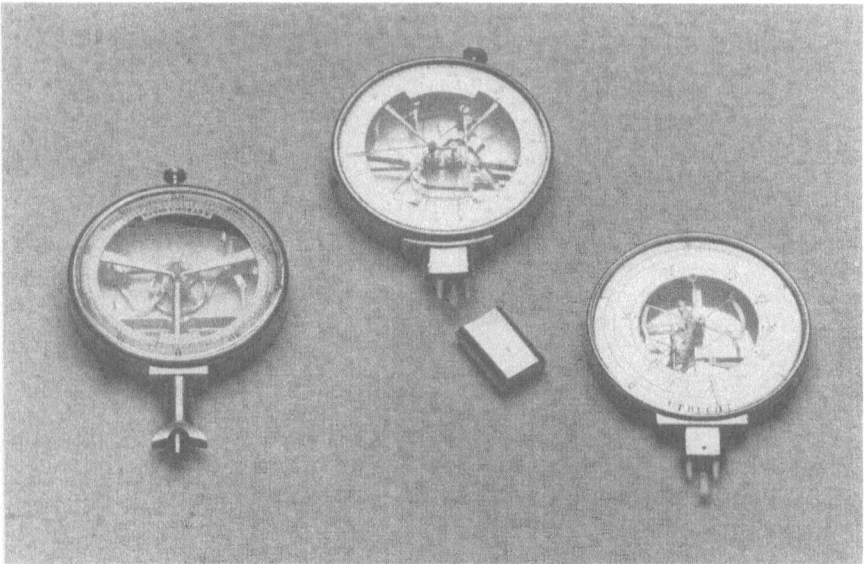

Fig. 3. (Left) Donders' tonometer of 1865 constructed by Stroh (London); (center) tonometer of Monnik, model I (1868); (right) model II constructed in the same year.

Since a reliable tonometer was still lacking, Monnik, a student under Donders and later trainee of Donders and Snellen, tried again and developed in 1868 a new type of tonometer (Fig. 3, center). He understood that he had to avoid one stumbling block. That was the fact that in most tonometers built before, the reference point for measuring the depth of the indentation of the sclera was the instant at which the edge of the tube touched the sclera. (As local anaesthesia of the cornea was yet unknown, scleral measurements were the only possibility). Monnik tried to solve this problem by using two small pins instead of a tube. Both pins were connected to one of the pointers. The central rod which exerted the scleral impression was connected with the second pointer. The difference in position of the two pointers indicated the depth of the indentation.

In his first model, Monnik had used a given force and determined the resulting depth of the indentation. But later he hoped to obtain better results if he measured the force required to reach a given depth of indentation. This idea he realized in his second model (Fig. 3, right). Even this instrument, however, was not a solution of the problem since its handling required too much attention and practice because both pointers as well as the positioning of the instrument upon the eye had to be observed at the same time. Nevertheless, in the hands of Donders, this instrument enabled him to discover that intraocular pressure is not increased during accommodation.

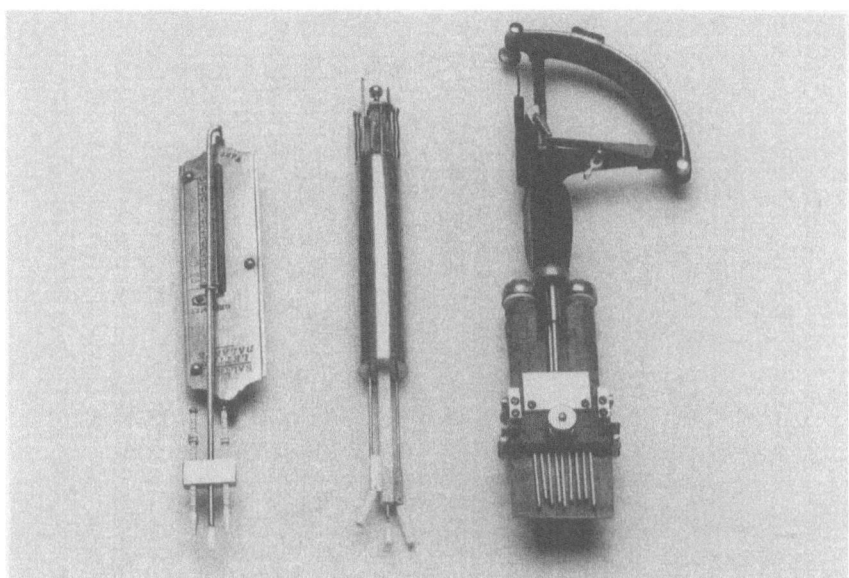

Fig. 4. (Left) tonomoter of Snellen, model I (1868); (center) Snellen's second model developed in 1872; (right) tonometer of Dor/Snellen of 1900.

In the same year, 1868, Donders' closest co-worker, Snellen, also developed a tonometer (Fig. 4, left). In his opinion, the depth of the scleral indentation alone was not reliable enough; also its shape should be taken into account. In his first model the indentation was produced by the pressure of a central rod exerted by the spring of a letter-balance. In addition, three pins were attached on either side of the central rod which moved independently of each other. Yet, although this arrangement indeed indicated the change in the shape of the indented sclera, the side pins slipped out too easily. Moreover, when the instrument was removed from the eye, the pins adhered to the sclera and slipped out further. The model illustrated here differs from the published prototype in that there is only one pin on either side of the central rod. The prototype published by Snellen is not present in the Utrecht instrument collection.

In Snellen's second prototype of 1872 the side pins could be fixed (Fig. 4, center). After he failed to relate the changes produced in the shape of the indented sclera with the intraocular tension, he gave up for the time being declaring that in his opinion, palpation was still the best method available to determine the intraocular pressure in ophthalmic practice!

Several tonometers were published since that time (Priestly Smith, 1879/ 1887; Maklakoff, 1885; Fick, 1888; Koster, 1895) but only the Maklakoff

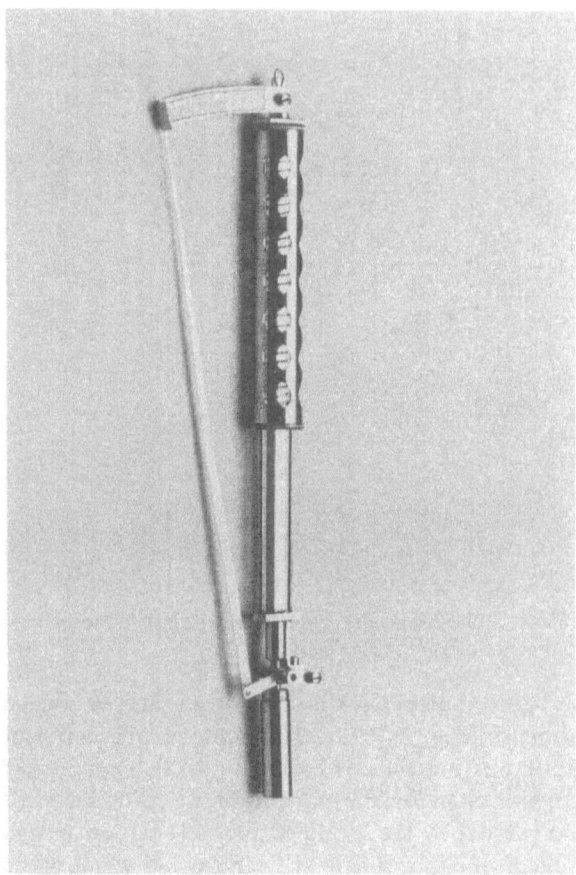

Fig. 5. Applanation tonometer of Seeuwen (1901).

applanation tonometer was successful and has been in use ever since in many countries.

In the meantime, Snellen had not abandoned the idea of constructing an overall reliable tonometer. In 1900 the original tonometer of Dor/Lecoultre (see above) was reconstructed (Fig. 4, right). The central rod which exerted pressure upon the eye produced a change in scleral shape, which change could be determined by the position of the side pins, as in Snellen's earlier model. Here, however, an electric relay could fix the pins in position. Yet as with his earlier models, even this instrument did not meet the necessary requirements for accurate measurement in ophthalmic practice (Seeuwen, 1901).

Also at the end of the 19th century, again a trainee of the Utrecht clinic, Seeuwen, designed a tonometer based upon the applanation principle (Fig. 5). The instrument was suspended above the eye. Though Seeuwen's concept was sound, the instrument was too difficult to handle and thus did not find its way into the daily practice.

Of all the tonometers constructed in the second half of the last century, only those that worked upon the applanation principle proved successful. But in ophthalmic practice, only the Maklakoff tonometer survived up to the present time as a clinically reliable instrument. None of the impression tonometers which were developed in the period from 1850 to 1900 was successful. One had to wait till 1905 when eventually Schiøtz published the design of his famous tonometer. For decades it set the trend in large areas of the ophthalmic world until Goldmann designed his world-wide accepted applanation tonometer (1954).

The Utrecht school has played in the 19th century a prominent role in the development of tonometry although it did not achieve the ultimate goal. The various impression tonometers designed and constructed by Donders, Snellen and their co-workers in the second half of the last century, although they were not a success in clinical practice, were nevertheless guiding and helping to show the way by trial and error to final success. Moreover, these efforts demonstrate not only the need which was felt for such an instrument but they also show the perseverance of the designers and researchers and last, not least, the high quality of the instrumentmakers of that period.

References

Donders FC. Über einen Spannungsmesser des Auges (letter from FC Donders to A von Graefe). Graefes Arch Ophthal 1863; 9: 215–221.
Dor H. Über ein verbessertes Tonometer. Zehenders Mbl Augenheil 1865; 3: 351–355.
Draeger J. Geschichte der Tonometrie. Basel: Karger, 1961.
Draeger J, Schweitzer NMJ. Über einige sehr alte Tonometer. Ophthalmologica 1962; 144: 221–228.
Fick A. Über Messung des Druckes im Auge. Pflügers Arch ges Physiol 1888; 42: 86.
Goldmann (1954) Ophthalmologica 109: 71.
Koster W. Beiträge zur Tonometrie und Manometrie des Auges. Graefes Arch Ophthal 1895; 41: 113–158.
Maklakoff A. L'Ophtalmotonometrie. Arch Ophtal Paris 1885; 5: 159–165.
Monnik AJW. Tonometers en tonometrie. Utrecht: Kemink, 1868.
Schiøtz HJ. Ein neues Tonometer. Arch Augenheilk 1905; 52: 401–424.
Smith P. A new tonometer. Ophth Rev 1887; 6: 32–42.
Snellen H, Landolt E. Optometrologie. Die Funktionsprüfungen des Auges, Ophthalmotonometrie. Graefe-Saemisch Handbuch ges Augenheilk. 1874; 1 Aufl 3: 185–194.
Seeuwen JJS. Iets over ophthalmotonometrie. Utrecht: Van de Weyer, 1901.

Address for offprints: Royal Netherlands Ophthalmic Hospital, F.C. Dondersstraat 65, 3572 JE Utrecht, the Netherlands

Documenta Ophthalmologica 68: 65–69 (1988)

The Utrecht Ophthalmic Hospital and the development of the ophthalmoscope

ISOLDE DEN TONKELAAR,[1] HAROLD E. HENKES[2] & GIJSBERT K. VAN LEERSUM[1]
[1] Royal Netherlands Ophthalmic Hospital, Utrecht, the Netherlands; [2] Department of Ophthalmology, Erasmus University Rotterdam, the Netherlands

Abstract. The first useful table model ophthalmoscope was designed by Donders and the instrumentmaker Epkens. With the use of this instrument Donders' pupil Van Trigt made the first drawings of the normal and pathological fundus of the eye. His contribution was of great importance for the early diffusion of knowledge of the fundus of the eye.

The invention of the ophthalmoscope by Helmholtz in 1851 was of great importance for the development of ophthalmology in general and for the history of ophthalmology in the city of Utrecht in particular, as F.C. Donders' (1818–1889) decision to become an ophthalmologist was greatly influenced by the invention of this instrument. Until then Donders had only shown interest in the physiology and pathophysiology of the eye, not especially in clinical problems. After a visit to London and Paris, where he met several famous ophthalmologists of that time (William Bowman, Friedrich von Jaeger, Albrecht von Graefe, Julius Sichel and Louis Auguste Desmarres), Donders announced that he was prepared to see patients. In an autobiographical speech he mentioned that a direct relation existed between his decision and the fact that the ophthalmoscope of Helmholtz became available one month earlier [1]. When the news of the new instrument spread, there was a run of patients who wished to be examined with the ophthalmoscope. Donders opened, at his own expense, a small policlinic for eye diseases, which lead to the foundation of the "Nederlands Gasthuis voor Ooglijders" (Netherlands Ophthalmic Hospital) in 1858 [1].

In 1851 Donders ordered an ophthalmoscope through Helmholtz. But Rekoss, Helmholtz's instrumentmaker in Königsberg, was unable to supply the ophthalmoscope in time. Before Donders received the instrument, the impatient man had already commissioned Epkens, an instrumentmaker in Amsterdam with the construction of a table model ophthalmoscope [2], designed to facilitate the drawing of fundus pictures (Fig. 1) [5]. It was the first model of its kind. In contrast to the instrument of Helmholtz, in which three superimposed glass plates were used, that partly reflected and partly

66

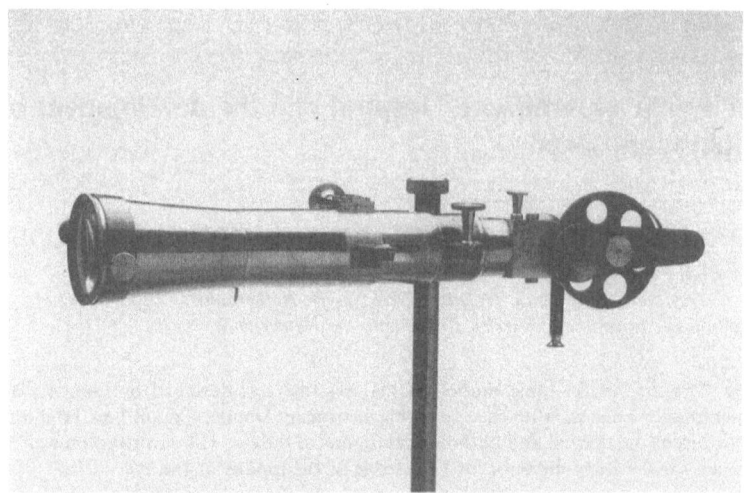

Fig. 1. Ophthalmoscope of Donders-Epkens (Model 3) (1852).

transmitted the light [3], the ophthalmoscope of Donders-Epkens was fit with a plane mirror with a central opening. The use of a mirror was an improvement because the intensity of illumination was considerably increased, but unfortunately, the polarisation effect of the glass plates had disappeared,

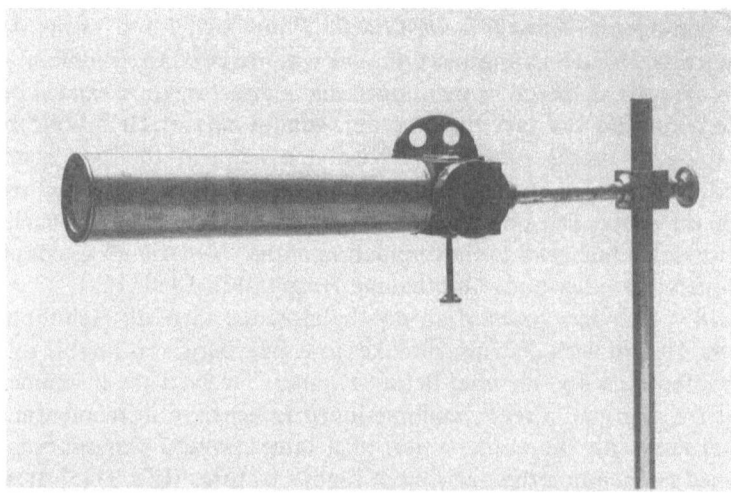

Fig. 2. Ophthalmoscope of Donders-Epkens (Model 1) (1851 or 1852).

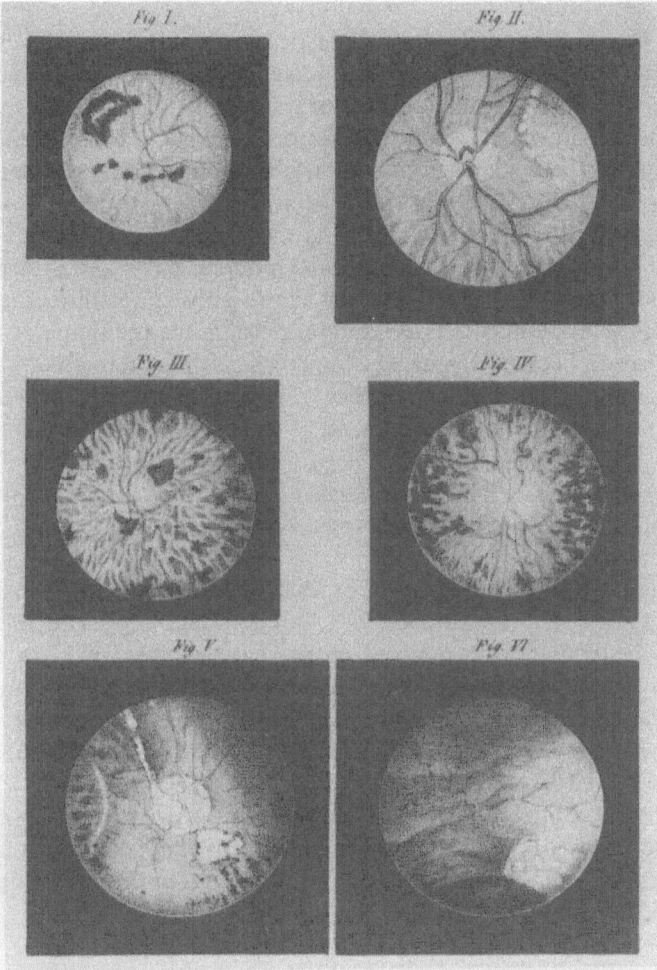

Fig. 3. Drawings of the fundus of the eye in Van Trigt's thesis (1853), showing a.o. a retinitis pigmentosa (Fig. IV) and a retinal detachment (Fig. VI).

which caused hindrance due to the reflection of the cornea [2]. A micrometer forms part of the instrument. The image of the micrometer on the fundus enabled the measurement of the details of the fundus. Both this instrument and the second model of Helmholtz's ophthalmoscope were equipped with a Rekoss disk and both were constructed for direct ophthalmoscopy [4].

A precursor of the ophthalmoscope of Donders-Epkens (Fig. 2), as well as the final instrument (Fig. 1) are present in the museum of the Royal Netherlands Ophthalmic Hospital. To our knowledge this precursor (Model

1) has not been published. It is less sophisticated than the final model (Model 3). The tube doesn't widen and the diameter of the opening through which the light passes is much smaller. Caps to screen the light from the eye of the patient and the investigator are not yet present, but a Rekoss disk forms already part of the instrument as well as a small bar which enables to turn the mirror slightly. There may have been a third instrument (Model 2), which, in case it did exist, must have been almost identical to the final model. A.C. Van Trigt (1825–1864), a pupil of Donders, published a design of a table model ophthalmoscope [5] which shows only minor differences compared with the final model. These differences concern the shape of the tube and the position of the micrometer. However, it is difficult to ascertain which model was first: the one that corresponds with the design of Van Trigt (Model 2) or the one we called the final model (Model 3). According to Snellen [6] Epkens delivered only one workable instrument. Therefore it is very likely that Model 2 has only existed in design. It also means that the instrument in the collection of the Royal Netherlands Ophthalmic Hospital is a unique specimen.

Van Trigt published the design of Model 2 in his thesis about the ophthalmoscope, called "De Speculo Oculi". Donders had suggested this timely subject to his trainee who received on the basis of this work the doctor's degree magna cum laude in 1853. In his thesis we find the first drawings of the fundus of the eye ever published, viz. a.o. a drawing of a retinitis pigmentosa (Fig. 3) (Table 3, Fig. IV) and of a retinal detachment (Fig. 3) (Table 3, Fig. VI) (Note 1).

Though the contribution of the Utrecht school to the development of ophthalmoscopy was limited to the invention of the Donders-Epkens ophthalmoscope, Van Trigt made a basic contribution to the knowledge of the diseases of the fundus of the eye.

Note

1. We should like to thank Drs. R. Hofman for his translation of the Latin text.

References

1. Donders FC. Autobiography. In: Het jubileum van professor F.C. Donders, gevierd te Utrecht op 27 en 28 mei 1888. Utrecht: Van de Weijer, 1889; 115–134.
2. Doesschate G ten. Een eeuw ophthalmoscopie. NTVG, 1952, 96 ii 14, p. 4–10.
3. Helmholtz H. Beschreibung eines Augen-Spiegels. Berlin: Förstner'sche Verlagsbuchhandlung, 1851.

4. Rucker CW. A history of the ophthalmoscope, Whiting printers and stationers, Rochester, Minnesota, 1971.
5. Trigt AC van. De speculo oculi. Diss. Utrecht: Van der Weijer, 1853.
6. Snellen H. Een halve eeuw oogspiegel. NTVG I, 1902; 306–314.

Address for offprints: Royal Netherlands Ophthalmic Hospital, F.C. Dondersstraat 65, 3572 JE Utrecht, the Netherlands

Documenta Ophthalmologica 68: 71–77 (1988)
© Kluwer Academic Publishers, Dordrecht

The foundation of experimental ophthalmology by Theodor Leber

WOLFGANG JAEGER

The University Eye Clinic, Bergheimer Str. 20, D-6900 Heidelberg, BRD

Abstract. Theodor Leber grew up in Heidelberg as the son of a professor of Romance languages. Initially he planned to study natural sciences. Bunsen's advice led him to medicine. During his studies he succeeded in solving a competition problem posed by Helmholtz in the medical department. A short period of practical work in the eye hospital of Knapp was unsatisfactory. In Vienna with the physiologist Carl Ludwig, he was able in 1863/64, at the age of only 24 years, to demonstrate the blood circulation of the eye by color injections into the arteries and veins. Since that time the schematic drawings of his results can be found in every textbook of ophthalmology. On the occasion of the congress of the German Ophthalmological Society in Heidelberg in 1864, Theodor Leber reported on these findings and met with immense approval. In 1864–67 he followed an invitation as coworker of Liebreich to Paris; in 1867 he became A.v. Graefe's coworker in Berlin; in 1871 he moved to Göttingen, which became the first eye clinic with a laboratory for experimental investigations.

The second epoch-making discovery accomplished by Leber was the detection of the fluid exchange in the eye. These results have also been confirmed by modern methods. Therefore, Theodor Leber can be called the father of experimental ophthalmology.

In his address of 1896 on the occasion of receiving the *von Graefe Medal* Leber said: "*I have had much fortune and success as an eye doctor, but, nevertheless, I am not a genuine ophthalmologist. The research, which I believe to be my best, belongs to the field of biology, and the eye just served as an extremely suitable object for research. What stimulates me to do research work are the rules of the living organisms. What satisfied me is to acquire information on the nature and connection of pathologic conditions.*"

After the invention of the ophthalmoscope by Helmholtz in 1850, clinical ophthalmology developed at an admirable speed. This was due to the fact that ingenious clinicians like Graefe, Donders, Bowman, Arlt and Liebreich developed ophthalmology to an independent clinical specialty.

During these first years little time was left for experimental research.

The abundance of diseases detected with the ophthalmoscope was so overwhelming that the ophthalmologists were kept busy during this first decade of modern ophthalmology.

Of course, such an ingenious observer as A.v. Graefe realized that the basic knowledge on which clinical decisions were based was not sufficient.

For this reason not only A.v. Graefe, but all participants of the congress of the Heidelberg Ophthalmological Society in September 1864 were fascinated by a lecture held by Theodor Leber, a 24-year-old and until then completely unknown young man, on the subject of *"Blood circulation of the eye."*

Leber wrote in his diary: *"I demonstrated some specimens serving as illustrations for the lecture and earned great applause. Later on, I had the chance to demonstrate them to Prof. v. Graefe and to Donders. Shortly before my departure for Paris I also showed them to Helmholtz."*

This lecture made Theodor Leber famous overnight.

Even during this congress he was asked by Liebreich to become his assistant in Paris. v. Graefe asked him to publish this lecture not only in the congress report, but also in extended form in the Archiv für Ophthalmologie which he had recently founded.

Helmholtz asked Leber, when he was already in Paris, through his father, if he wanted to work in his institute of physiology in Heidelberg. Only a short time later Graefe wrote Leber, who was still in Paris, inviting him to become his assistant in Berlin.

Everyone who heard Theodor Leber's lecture on the 4th of September 1864 might have felt that a breakthrough had happened: the foundation of a new discipline: experimental ophthalmology.

Who was this 24-year-old, unknown Theodor Leber?

Theodor Leber was born on the 29th of February 1840 in Karslruhe, a date which caused much fun on the occasion of birthday congratulations. His father was a highly respected college professor whose field was Romance languages. Theodor's mother died early, but his father did everything possible to educate Theodor and his two brothers in the best possible way. During frequent strolls with his father through the fields and woods, Theodor's interest in the natural sciences soon became apparent. Learning was easy for Theodor and at the age of 17 he was ready to enter the university. On his graduation report it says: *"Theodor will study the natural sciences."* But actually he was quite undecided which avenue he should pursue. His interests were numerous. Botany and, later, chemistry were his first choices. Only after his father had received a warning from the famous professor of chemistry, Bunsen, *"alas, there are so many chemists and so few positions,"* did Leber decide to study medicine, which seemed to offer better prospects for economic security. As a medical student he participated in a contest by Helmholtz to establish the relationship between performance and fatigue of muscles. This was, of course, almost too ambitious an undertaking for the young student whose background seemed quite inadequate for such a study. But with intensive work and determination he was able to win the first prize,

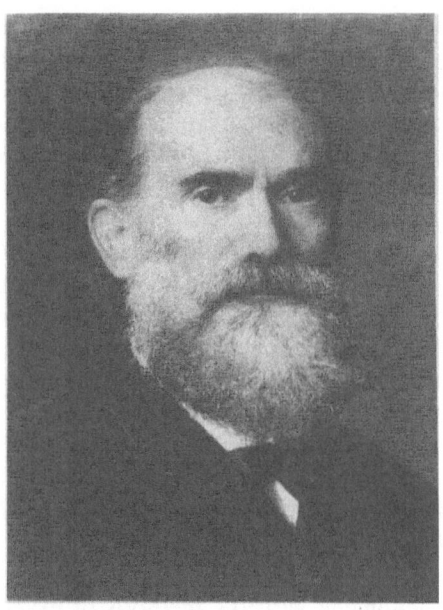

Fig. 1. Theodor Leber (1840–1917).

even over the apparently better prepared contestant, Kronecker, who later became professor of physiology at the University of Bern.

After having received his degree, Leber's first contacts with ophthalmology were during the year he spent as an assistant to Jakob Herman Knapp, who had founded a flourishing private eye hospital and was an associate professor at the University of Heidelberg.

But the short association with Knapp did not swing young Leber toward ophthalmology. He was attracted to the field of physiology because, in his opinion, it offered a more scientific approach to problems. He felt that ophthalmology in the way Knapp practiced it, was directed more toward the practical application of known facts than to basic research.

Therefore, he decided in 1863 to abandon his position in the hospital of Knapp in order to continue experimental studies in an institute of physiology. Despite his great admiration for Helmholtz, he had the feeling that Helmholtz in his ideas was already far beyond the goal he was looking for; he searched for a teacher who could instruct him on experimental work.

In the history of theoretical physics in the twenties of this century we can find a description paralleling these thoughts of Theodor Leber: Three important teachers existed in Germany: Max Planck, Albert Einstein and Arnold Sommerfeld. The description used a metaphor.

About Max Planck it was said that he showed the mountains in their monumental beauty, however, one could only admire them from the far distance. The genius of Albert Einstein still might be understood, but one would not be able to follow him from peak to peak. From Arnold Sommerfeld, however, one could learn to climb mountains and under his guidance one could finally manage even the most difficult climbs.

Helmholtz was comparable to Max Planck and Albert Einstein. Leber, however, was looking for someone to teach him "*to climb mountains.*"

He found such a teacher in Carl Ludwig at the Josephinum in Vienna. At first Ludwig did not want to accept him because the vacations were just about to begin and he was afraid not to be able to guide the young coworker as he wanted to. But then Ludwig cancelled his vacations and it is due to this coincidence that Theodor Leber found a teacher who gave him in this stage of his scientific development exactly what he needed.

Theodor Leber wrote to his father: "*I found in Prof. Ludwig an always friendly and cooperative teacher with sensitive and hard criticism, a master of experimental physiology.*"

Leber was enthusiastic about the way Ludwig emphasized the necessity to explore biological phenomena with the methods of exact research and to reduce them to rules which are also valid in physics and chemistry. Physiology ought to be the science of physics and chemistry applied to the living organism. Leber was so impressed by this enthusiastic spirit of his teacher that he himself spent most of his time in the laboratory.

Carl Ludwig had just developed a new method of injecting blood vessels in order to demonstrate the arteries and veins in the different organs of the body. Earlier experiments had been done with emulsions of small particles.

The new method is described by Theodor Leber himself: "*I used mixtures of glycerol with soluble Berlin blue as a blue substance and a solution of ferrocyanic copper in ammonia as a red substance. Sometimes I also used a mixture of glycerol with fine barit. Injections of glue were only used to demonstrate the big vessels. With these methods the injection of adult eyes is rather easy. Only the veins of the iris present difficulties. They are only in rare cases completely filled. Therefore, I used for this purpose the eyes of children. In these eyes the choroidal vessels are wider and, therefore, the injections easier. The injection of the iris is here also possible without difficulties.*

During the following preparations the glycerol is washed out of the vessels. Only the different colors remain in the walls of the vessels. Therefore, the vessels had their natural size."

Leber must have worked with unique energy during this year. Reading his letters and diaries from these months one is reminded of the famous words of the torero: "*Fuera todo el mondo.*"

Moreover, Leber had the fortune to have found a colleague in the institute who could paint his specimens in a masterly fashion. Those pictures found the way into all textbooks and handbooks of ophthalmology of the world as illustrations of the anatomy of ocular vessels and are still used today.

Leber summarized the results of his work in a few words: "*In the eye there are three vascular systems:*

1. The ciliary system, which supplies the sclera, choroid, ciliary body and iris; 2. The retinal system, which is exclusively reserved for the optic nerve and the retina; 3. The conjunctival system, which is found in all areas where the eye is protected by the conjunctiva. These three systems are not completely isolated from each other. There exist some connections. For instance, the retinal system is connected directly and indirectly with the ciliary system around the insertion of the optic nerve, and the conjunctival system is connected with the ciliary vessels at the corneal limbus. This illustration gives a schematic view of the different vessels within the eye." Norman Ashton succeeded in completing this work of Theodor Leber by using the modern neopren injections. He demonstrated even more subtle and fascinating details.

When Theodor Leber immediately, after the Heidelberg congress of 1864, went to Paris, he became a coworker of Liebreich. There he worked clinically as well as experimentally. Three years later (1867) he followed an invitation of Graefe to Berlin.

Leber characterized Graefe in the following way: "*Graefe was a master in intuitive understanding of the symptoms and the pathologic background of a disease. With all his energy he tried to find methods to fight the disease. His therapeutical genius led him to marvelous successes. I learned from him that clinical experience, observations on pathologic changes and experimental research complement each other mutually achieving a thorough understanding of complicated processes in the organism.*"

In 1869 Leber's habilitation was completed, just one year before Graefe's short life came to a tragic end.

As the successor of Graefe, Prof. Schweigger from Göttingen came to Berlin, Leber received an invitation to move to Göttingen, which at that time became the first eye clinic with an experimental laboratory.

Leber published his second research paper only three years later, which was also a breakthrough in the field of experimental ophthalmology.

In 1873 Theodor Leber published "*Studies on the fluid exchange in the eye.*" He refuted the generally accepted theory that Descemet's membrane was responsible for preventing the aqueous humor from infiltrating the corneal stroma. In an ingeniously simple experiment he demonstrated that the endothelium, not the membrane, actually controlled the flow of fluid from the anterior chamber into the cornea. The experiment was conducted

76

in the following way: Freshly excised corneas from cattle and horses were tightly mounted over one end of a U-shaped glass tube. The space directly beneath the cornea was filled with water and the rest of the tube filled with mercury. The water pressure on the cornea was changed and measured by simply varying and measuring the height of the mercury column.

More fluid penetrated an isolated Descemet's membrane in a shorter period of time after the endothelium had been brushed off than with the endothelium intact.

In an experiment on living rabbits, Leber entered the anterior chamber with a blunt hook and destroyed the endothelium in some areas by moving the hook over the posterior surface of the cornea. Within 15 minutes after this procedure, the corneal stroma became cloudy in places corresponding to the sites of injury. These results have all been confirmed in our time by other investigators. At the first congress of the German Ophthalmological Society after the Second World War in 1948 in Heidelberg, David Cogan gave a report on this confirmation of Leber's results with modern methods. The close connections of German and international ophthalmology were demonstrated on this example in an impressive way.

We may rightly say that Leber's findings 110 years ago established the fundamental facts of experimental ophthalmology. This opened the way to the understanding of many clinical phenomena.

Thus, while more elaborate and sophisticated methods in recent years provided more detailed insight into biological mechanisms, Leber accomplished the breakthrough more than 110 years ago.

Acknowledgement

As far as Theodor Leber's letters and diary are cited, these have been placed at my disposal by family-archives of Theodor Leber's family. For this possibility I should like to express my thanks.

References

1. Cogan D. Untersuchungen zur klinischen Physiologie der Hornhaut. Ber der Dt Ophth Ges 1949; 54: 6–13.
2. Hirschberg J. Theodor Leber. In: Graefe-Sämisch. Handbuch der gesamten Augenheilkunde, XV. BD., 2. Buch. Leipzig: Wilhelm Engelmann, 1918; 52–60.
3. Jaeger W. Theodor Lebers Elternhaus. Klin Mbl Augenheilk 1976; 168: 595–598.
4. Leber Th. Über den Einfluß mechanischer Arbeit auf die Ermüdung der Muskeln. Inaug Diss Heidelberg. Zeitschr f ration Medizin 3. Reihe, Bd. 18, 1863; 262–288.

5. Leber Th. Anatomische Untersuchungen über die Blutgefäße des menschlichen Auges. Wiener Akademie der Wissenschaften. Denkschriften der Mathematisch-Naturwissenschaftl. Klasse der Kaiserl. Akademie der Wissenschaften zu Wien. Bd. XXIV, 1865; 297–326. This epoch-making work of Theodor Leber will be published as facsimile in German as well as in English and French in: The Classics of Ophthalmology Library. The English translation has been undertaken by Irene Maumenee, the French translation by Pierre Amalric.

6. Leber Th. Studien über den Flüssigkeitswechsel im Auge. v Graefes Arch 1873; 29/2: 87–185.

7. Leber Th. Die Zirkulations- und Ernährungsverhältnisse des Auges. In Graefe-Sämisch, Handbuch der gesamten Augenheilkunde. 1. Aufl Bd II. Leipzig: Wilhelm Engelmann, 1876; 302–392.

8. Stocker FW, Reichle K. Theodor Leber and the Endothelium of the Cornea. Am J Ophth 1974; 78: 893–896.

Address for offprints: Prof. Dr. W. Jaeger, University Eye Hospital, Beigheimer Str. 20, D-6900 Heidelberg, BRD

Documenta Ophthalmologica 68: 79–103 (1988)
© Kluwer Academic Publishers, Dordrecht

Georg Joseph Beer: A review of his life and contributions*

DANIEL M. ALBERT[1] & FREDERICK C. BLODI[2]
[1]*Boston, Massachusetts; and* [2]*Iowa City, Iowa, USA*

Introduction

The establishment of ophthalmology as an independent scientific speciality came about largely through the efforts and example of Georg Joseph Beer in Vienna in the early nineteenth century. Beer was outstanding in his clinical practice of ophthalmology and surgery, as a teacher and as an author. He was the founder of the first ophthalmological school and clinic. His greatest text was his *Lehre von den Augenkrankheiten*, the first volume of which appeared in 1813 and the second in 1817. In 1819, George C. Monteath translated and edited the work. For the English-speaking physician this translation remains the finest testament to Georg Beer's genius and perception.

The only comprehensive review of Beer's life and contributions is that by Hirschberg and this has recently been made available in the English language as a result of Blodi's translation. Most of the material that follows is drawn from this source.

Georg Joseph Beer's background and career

Georg Joseph Beer was born in Vienna on December 23, 1763, in the former Königin-Kloster (Queen's Convent) at the Joseph Palace, where his father was the administrator (Fig. 1). Hirschberg notes that Georg Beer came from a modest family and "had to fight poverty, worry, and persecution. This left a scar in his personality which manifests itself in some detail even when he was a middle-aged man." Hirschberg states that his father vowed at the time of his son's birth that Georg would enter the priesthood. During his formative years, however, he showed strong interest in music, painting, and in observing nature. His father died when Georg was 15 years old and the son

*Much of the material presented here previously appeared in the "Notes" accompanying the facsimile edition of Monteath's translation of Beer's *Lehre von den Augenkrankheiten* published by Gryphon Editions in 1985. This is reprinted with the permission of the publisher.

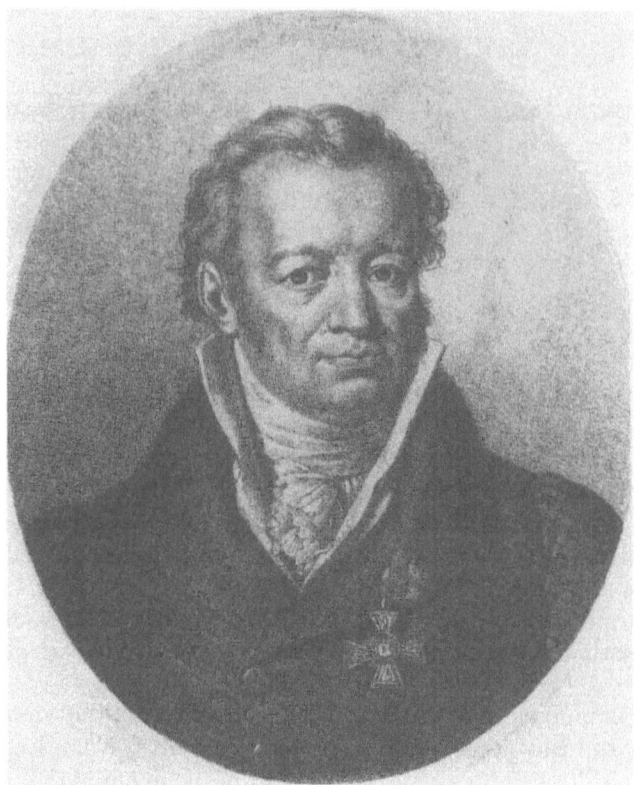

Fig. 1. Portrait of Georg Joseph Beer as professor of ophthalmology in Vienna.

then became responsible for the care of his mother and his siblings. His artistic talents led him to enroll in the School of Painting of the Academy of Fine Arts and its curator was sufficiently impressed with Beer's talents to propose that he travel to Rome to study art. Beer's love of art, however, was exceeded by his interest in medicine and he undertook his medical studies instead.

In order to appreciate Beer's role in the establishment of the Viennese School of Ophthalmology, it is necessary to review certain other aspects of ophthalmic history in Austria. In the late 18th century, Baron Michael de Wenzel was one of the most prominent ophthalmic surgeons in Europe. Although accounts vary, it appears that Wenzel attained great skill as an itinerant coucher of cataracts. Wenzel subsequently improved Daviel's method of cataract extraction and rejected couching completely. His methods were recorded by his son, Jakob de Wenzel, in his *Traité de la Cataracte* published in 1786. The story is told that a lady of the court of the Empress Maria Theresa lost her vision from cataracts and none of the local oculists dared to operate on her. The Empress consequently invited Baron Wenzel to treat the woman, and he did so with a successful result. The Empress, chagrined at the poor state of ophthalmology in Austria, asked Baron Wenzel to instruct Joseph Barth (1743–1818) in ophthalmic surgery.

Barth, a native of Malta, subsequently became Professor of Surgery and Ophthalmology in Vienna in 1773. Emperor Joseph II also considered it undesirable for Austria to be dependent on foreign surgeons and drew up a contract with Barth. The latter was directed to train two oculists for the Imperial States. The first of these was Ehrenritter who died in 1790. The second, Johann Adam Schmidt (1759–1809), went on to become Associate Professor of Anatomy and Surgery at the Joseph's Academy in 1788. Although an ophthalmologist of international standing, he nevertheless failed to establish an ophthalmological school in Vienna. A third student of Barth's, Georg P. Prochaska, practiced in Prague. On Barth's retirement in 1791 he was called back to Vienna and was an instructor in ophthalmology until 1818.

Georg Joseph Beer attracted the attention of Joseph Barth as a medical student. Barth recognized his talents as an anatomical illustrator and for seven years engaged him to record the details of Barth's dissections. Barth published a textbook on the anatomy of the muscles in 1786 (republished in a posthumous second edition in 1819) which includes beautiful illustrations of the ocular muscles. Although the artist is not identified, Hirschberg suspects that Beer contributed to this work. Barth refused to act as ophthalmic teacher to the studious Beer who graduated from the University of Vienna in 1786 at the age of 23 years with a Doctor of Medicine degree. Even after his graduation, Beer continued to work as an anatomical illustrator for Barth, hoping vainly for a change in heart by the latter. Beer referred to his years of apprenticeship with Barth as his "years of torture." Barth, in fact, refused to give any assistance to his young assistant in gaining a career in ophthalmology. When Beer was 36 years of age he wrote that "Barth was insufferable as a chief; his arrogance and despotism alienated every subalternate employee who was not willing to kiss his boots." Hirschberg notes that Beer was "brusquely, even brutally, rejected. The two broke completely. Beer started as a general practitioner and elected — to the complete surprise of Barth — ophthalmology as his specialty. He also married at that time."

It is sometimes stated that Beer was heir to the surgical wizardry of Baron Wenzel and Joseph Barth. The truth of the matter is that Beer was his own teacher in ophthalmology. Pillat has correctly stressed that Beer was "a self-made man."

Hirschberg records that Arlt apparently told Ernst Fuchs that Beer had participated when Wenzel originally instructed Barth. Hirschberg points out that this is impossible because in 1778 Beer was only 15 years old. He further states that Beer as a medical student learned from Professor Barth only what Barth wanted to show and tell the student. He notes however, "We can assume . . . as Arlt tells us, that Beer assisted Professor Barth when he operated each springtime on a number of indigent cataract patients as he was obliged to do."

Beer's student, assistant, and eventually successor to his chair in Vienna, Anton Rosas (1791–1855) maintained that Beer was the third pupil of Barth. This, however, is inconsistent with Beer's own account. Johann Adam Schmidt pointedly mentioned in his lectures that Barth had instructed only two men, Prochaska and Schmidt himself. Of the ensuing bitterness, Hirschberg writes: "Barth and Schmidt tried to crush Beer; they denied that Beer had any capabilities as an ophthalmologist because he had not been the pupil of a master; nevertheless, Beer was already a licensed ophthalmologist and developed into a master of the field on the basis of his own talents. This scenario reminds one of Wagner's *Meistersinger* where the apprentice also overtakes the teacher."

Beer himself wrote, "Soon thereafter I was involved in disputes; one tried to offend me and to rob me of the confidence of the public; one attempted to damage my practice of ophthalmology before I had become a licensed physician. I had to be extremely careful and I did not accept dubious cases. I worked with limitless diligence on every patient and hoped for a fortunate outcome. Any unfortunate outcome of an ocular disease, even completely without my fault, would certainly have led to my downfall because my enemies, or more specifically, enemy, followed each of my steps with great scrutiny." In 1786, the year of Beer's graduation, he opened an ophthalmic private practice and set up two rooms in his apartment for the treament of indigent patients. Beer described this facility in his book, *Das Auge*, as follows: "My private eye institute consisted of two spacious rooms in my apartment. I admit there every year those poor cataract patients who come to me during May and June referred from one of the provincial governments for an eye operation on an indigent basis. I also admit those eye patients who suffer from a dangerous disease which needs emergency treatment and constant medical care. These patients stay with me at my own expense and are cared for just like a paying patient. Many eyes would be lost if I referred these patients to the General Hospital and waited until they could be admitted, which usually takes one or several days." As indicated in Beer's statement, he administered his eye institute for the first twenty years without any outside support.

Professor Erna Lesky interprets the modest and unofficial style of Beer's institute as follows: "Before the new specialty (i.e. ophthalmology) was deemed worthy of teaching, its efficiency and value had to be tested in gratuitous treatment of the poor. Hence it was in the field of social welfare that the new specialty received its official recognition: in 1806 the government established in Vienna a separate ophthalmic outpatients' department for indigent patients and Beer was appointed the first social welfare ophthalmologist with a salary of 400 florins."

By 1806, in fact, Beer's reputation as an ophthalmologist and teacher was considerable. In 1798, he led a scientific program at the opening of the second Practical Private Course on Ocular Diseases and in 1802 became an associate professor at the University.

Rivalries, jealousies and other adversities that Beer faced at the time are succinctly summarized by Lesky as follows: "It was much more difficult to establish the new specialty as a subject of instruction. In 1797 Beer suggested to the government the establishment of an eye clinic at the General Hospital where hitherto he had been allowed to carry out cataract operations in the months of May and June only. In 1798, he published in the Salzburg Medical-Surgical Journal a detailed plan for an eye clinic. In spite of the general approval which the plan received from outside, it was rejected by the faculty as well as the government, together with similar plans which the stubborn man submitted in 1805 and 1807. Indeed, in 1809 he was also turned down when he proposed to train two oculists against an inclusive fee of 500 florins per annum (Barth's fee had been 1000 florins). Highly influential new adversaries had arisen against Beer. The faculty's disapproval was obviously influenced by the physiologist Georg Prochaska (1749–1820), who was himself an oculist in much demand and since the departure of his teacher Barth, i.e. since 1791, had been teaching ophthalmology in conjunction with advanced anatomy. He now feared that the creation of a separate Chair of Ophthalmology might cause him the loss of the ophthalmological part of his teaching job. This part was, in fact, taken from him when the Chair of Ophthalmology was raised to a Chair in Ordinary, in 1818. At court, Beer's adversary was the Protomedicus himself. It was incompatible with Stifft's conservative outlook that the Vienna master of ophthalmology professed natural-philosophical ideas and was, in addition a zealous member of the Society of Physicians which had been harboring a passionate spirit intent on medical innovation since the time of the Franks, senior and junior. In 1812, Beer was nevertheless appointed professor and a separate clinic for ophthalmology was established, one of the main reasons for this being that the Protomedicus still preferred the natural-philosophy inclined Beer to Johann Nepomuk Rust who was aspiring to the chair in ophthalmology and whose operational daring was repugnant to Stifft."

The official decrees about the establishment of lectures in ophthalmology and about the appointment of Beer read as follows:

I. "Following a decree of the government of April 15 of this year his Majesty has ordered the following in order to regulate the study of ophthalmology.

This should be inititated with the beginning of the next school year in all universities where a full professor of ophthalmology is already appointed, as well as at the University of Vienna. It should be initiated in all other universities as soon as a full professor of ophthalmology can be appointed:

1. A complete course on theoretical and practical ophthalmology has to be given in every semester so that in each school year two such full courses will be available.
2. For fifth year medical students a one semester course on ophthalmology is obligatory.
3. The students of surgery are not obligated to study ophthalmology, but they are permitted to attend these lectures and demonstrations on a voluntary basis.
4. These lectures should last one hour, five days of the week.
5. Those who would like to take the rigorous examination in ophthalmology and would like to obtain a diploma for an ophthalmologist have to prove that they have attended two semester courses and that they have performed one cataract operation under the supervision of a professor.
6. Students of surgery can be admitted to these two courses of ophthalmology only when they have completed their surgical studies.
7. The lectures on this branch of medicine will be held in the language of the country.
8. Each university has to establish a clinical institute for ophthalmology, as it exists for medicine and surgery, which should be established in the hospital in which during the entire school year eye patients will be admitted and close to which the lectures will be held.

Pr. Gr. Lazansky Stlrt. m.p.
Member of the Imperial Royal Study Commission
Vienna, March 2, 1818
v. Cavallar m.p.

II. In regard to the decree of May 2, No. 60 in which the government expresses its intention as far the teaching of ophthalmology at this university is concerned: Upon the recommendation from highest authority it is therefore ordered that a special professorship for this branch of medicine will be established at the University of Vienna and in Prague. This decree is based on the order of May 2 of this year following the decision by the Emperor of August 3.

According to my cabinet decree of April 22, 1818, the instruction of ophthalmology has to begin with the next school year; Dr. Beer will accord-ing to my decision of March 25, 1812 be appointed full professor with an annual stipend of 2,000 florins.

The professor of ophthalmology will receive all the rights of a full chair-man which up to now was occupied by the professor of physiology who also taught ophthalmology; the latter will in the future not teach ophthalmology any more.

We therefore will appoint the associate professor Br. Beer to full professor and the government will initiate the necessary steps to fulfill the decision of the Emperor.

The Imperial Royal Study Commission
Vienna, August 13, 1818.

Thus, by these two special decrees, an eye department was founded in the General Hospital of Vienna and Beer was named its director and also made extraordinary professor.

During the first five years of Beer's private eye institute's existence, 1587 patients were admitted and subsequently transferred to the orphanage, the General Hospital, the work house, or the Jewish Hospital. The institute was in fact an outpatient clinic. One hundred fifty four operations were perfor-med during this time, of which 124 were reported to be successful. During the ensuing six years, this facility became the birthplace of ophthalmology in Europe. Beer began his lectures in his capacity as professor on April 28, 1812, and his clinic in the General Hospital of Vienna began to function on January 19, 1813. The eye deparment continues in operation to this day, on the second floor of the Fourth Court of the General Hospital of Vienna.

This clinic consisted of three spacious rooms, the largest of which was used for lectures and surgery. It held 150 students, was well lighted and neatly painted green. According to Juengken it contained portraits of Barth and Lefebure; a small but well chosen library; a collection of pathologic and anatomic preparations of the eye (apparently the only such collection in existence at that time); and a collection of eye instruments some of which came from as far away as India. The remaining two rooms, also painted green, served as wards and contained eight to twelve beds. A salaried assistant, residing in the hospital, was assigned to the clinic. Beer worked with this assistant and with his son-in-law Friedrich Jaeger. In the morning Beer gave public lectures and in the afternoon taught privately in his house, discussing the indigent eye patients.

Ophthalmology was made a compulsory subject for the medical student with five hours of weekly lecture given for one semester being the minimum requirement, as indicated in the first official decree. By all accounts, Beer was an extremely popular teacher.

Reports of Beer's skill as a surgeon were generally favorable. Weller stated that it was a pleasure to watch Beer perform difficult cataract operations. Chelius referred to Beer's "unexcelled skill as a surgeon." W. Soemmering wrote, "Professor Beer performs with his peculiar skill and ease the corneal incision." Mackenzie in 1818 lauded Beer's "profundity and amazing dexterity." In the same year Juengken noted, however, "Through his hand trembled somewhat, he guided the knife securely and gently, only slowly so that aqueous escaped."

The following statistics are taken from the *Vierte Übersicht aller Vorfälle in dem Oeffent. klin. Institut für d. Augenkrankheiten, a.d.k.k. Universität in Wien* (Fourth review of all events in the public clinical institute for eye diseases at the Imperial Royal University of Vienna), by Proffessor Beer (1816): "There were 106 eye patients admitted (between November 4, 1815 and September 7, 1816) and there were 158 outpatients. There were 54 cataract patients and 35 of these were operated on in front of students, 28 with complete success. The number of students was in the first semester 77, in the second semester 93, together 170, among them were 91 foreigners. Dr. Brosse of Riga, Dr. Faber of Graz and the doctor and ophthalmologist Friedrich Jaeger from Hohenlohe performed publicly in the clinic cataract operations with great success." Beer was described as a teacher with an open mind and open heart, quite in contrast to Professor Barth.

In 1819, Beer suffered a stroke which left him incapacitated and he died in Vienna in 1821. Contrary to expectations, his successor was not his most gifted pupil and son-in-law, Friedrich Jaeger, but rather the highly competent Anton Rosas. Rosas wrote the following words concerning Beer:

"Who would not know his great merits about our specialty to which he dedicated thirty years with his indefatigable diligence and with rare ambition? It is his constant ambition to improve ophthalmology on its way to a rational empiricism and perfection. He had a warm love for the welfare of mankind and therefore actively communicated to the entire world his knowledge and experience which he had acquired by laborious and difficult work. Many dogmas of our specialty which were previously known only to a small number of individuals became the common knowledge of all physicians: his keen ambition to stimulate all his students and to transmit to them a love for our specialty; his instructive and comprehensive bedside teaching; his supportive attitude toward all patients who came to him for help and his consolations for those who experienced misfortune; his more than 1800 sucessful cataract operations; his numerous informative monographs about eye diseases; all these are facts which must secure for him the deepest admiration and the warmest gratitude of his contemporaries and of all posterity."

Georg Joseph Beer's major contributions to ophthalmology

As noted in the above discussion of Beer's life, in 1786 he founded the first private eye hospital in history which consisted of two rooms in his own apartment. His services were provided free to the poor. In 1812 by special decree of the Emperor, and as a result of Beer's efforts, an eye department was founded in the General Hospital of Vienna. Georg Joseph Beer was named its director and also made professor. He thus was founder of the Vienna School of Ophthalmology and through his teachings and writings was responsible for the establishment of "modern" ophthalmology as a recognized specialty in Austria and Germany and throughout Europe. We will now consider in more detail his contribution as a teacher, as an ophthalmic surgeon and clinician, and as an author.

Of Beer's numerous contributions to ophthalmology, his most profound impact on the specialty was as a teacher. The most influential ophthalmologists of the following generation were his pupils. These included Friedrich Jaeger, his assistant and later his son-in-law; Anton Rosas, his successor as professor of ophthalmology at the Imperial Royal University of Vienna; von Walther; C.F. Graefe; Textor; J.N. Fisher; K.M. Langenbeck; Chelius; Ammon; Weller; Ritterich; Dzondi; Benedikt; Flaerer; Albini; Fabini; Flemming; William Mackenzie of Glasgow; and George F. Frick of Baltimore. Although Beer quarrelled with many of his contemporaries, he appears to have been universally revered by his students.

Undoubtedly much of his appeal to his students and impact on them resulted from his being a unique role model as an ophthalmic specialist. After being fully trained in medicine and general surgery, he limited his practice to the treatment of diseases of the eye. He did this in an age when the medical community and the public associated specialization in the treament of eye diseases with the long tradition of itinerant quacks who had practiced under the appellation of "oculists." In reaction to this, distinguished individuals such as Benjamin Travers, Samuel Cooper, and even the medical historian A. Hirsch concluded that advances in the surgery of the eye could only be made by those who practiced surgery "in its entirety." But Beer, together with such great ophthalmologists as Brisseau, Maitre Jan, St. Yves, Daviel, Pellier de Quengsy, Richter and A.W. Andreae, proved this contention incorrect.

At the other extreme, Beer rejected the elitism of Barth, who had made his life so miserable, and Johann Adam Schmidt, who wrote, "I do not think highly of surgeons who have been trained in a school where the skills are not transmitted like hereditary traits."

The most important operation performed on the eye in Beer's time was cataract extraction, and here Beer was both an innovator and a master. Unlike the surgeons of previous generations who blindly clung to the old dogma about cataract that were found in Greek and Arabian texts, Beer for the most part based his practice and teaching on new anatomical concepts. He did, early on, persist in the idea of a "membranous cataract" as had been taught since the ninth century in Arabian medicine. This idea regarding the nature of cataracts was also accepted by Heister, Albrecht von Haller, Sharp, and Daviel. He came in time, however, to know the true nature of most cataracts, even giving the best description to that date of the hypermature, or Morgagnian cataract, first observed by Platner and given its more complete description by Morgagni.

During Beer's early years in medicine, dislocation of the cataract had become again quite popular, when in 1785 von Wullburg replaced the usual couching by reclination (i.e. dislodging the lens backwards). Scarpa in Italy became a staunch advocate of reclination. Beer noted in his *Repertorium* in 1799 that reclination was the best method of couching a cataract. Beer pointed out, however, that couching of a partially or totally solid cataract is only an apparent cure and gives transient or palliative relief. He realized that a cataract will never dissolve in the vitreous and reported finding on anatomical examinations a small lens in the eye even 20 years after the couching. He also noted an instance in one eye where he saw the lens rise again 30 years after it had been couched. Beer still thought, however, that there were special cases where couching had advantages over extraction.

As the dispute between extraction and couching of cataracts raged in Europe, discission or "needling" of the cataract became an important operation. Beer, through painful experience, came to realize that this operation should be performed only when the cataract is soft and the patient young. It also was indicated in certain medical conditions such as for patients with chronic cough, asthma, or those who could not lie on their back; but the results were of limited success. Hirschberg notes that in employing this operation on a series of 19 small children, Beer and F. Jaeger utilized almost all the principles of "modern" discission surgery. The only missing aspect was evacuation of the swollen lens matter in cases of secondary glaucoma. Ironically, although Beer introduced the irrigator to anterior segment surgery, he never adapted Guerin's method of irrigation of lens cortex.

Despite dabbling with reclination and discission, Beer recognized the importance of Daviel's cataract extraction and championed this procedure. He stated in his *Repertorium*, "How many thousand patients already praise the inventor of the cataract extraction and how many more will laud him in the future? . . . The thoughtful surgeons will always recognize the tremendous value of your discovery and many later generations will honor your memory and will think of you with reverence and gratitude."

Beer attempted to improve on Daviel's method. He stated in his *Methode den grauen Starr mit der Kapsel auszuziehen* . . . (Vienna, 1799) "If one extracts the cataract intracapsularly, then it is not necessary to introduce Daviel's spoon to remove cataract remnants; the healing is quicker, the visual acuity better, and the after-cataract is avoided. Disadvantages of the procedure are a certain propensity for prolapse of vitreous and iris."

Hirschberg collected the data from Beer's published reports on 58 eyes treated with intracapsular extraction and found the following results:

(1) " perfect" visual acuity after 43 extractions.

(2) "mediocre" visual acuity after 10 extractions.

(3) purulent infections after 5 extractions.

Hirschberg notes that the procedure Beer followed had been devised by G.A. Richter and reported by him in 1776 but that Beer never emphasized Richter's priority. He also recounts the acrimonious dispute that Beer's endorsement of the intracapsular led to with his competitor Johann Adam Schmidt. Beer's enthusiasm for the procedure continued and in 1799 in his *Repertorium* he stated that he "performs nearly always an intracapsular cataract extraction." Eighteen years later, however, in his 1817 edition of his *Augenkrankheiten* he stated, "if we are dealing with a cataract of medium consistency, i.e. neither too hard nor soft down to the nucleus, one can without fear attempt to perform an intracapsular cataract extraction according to my method which I published in 1799." However when Juengken visited Beer in 1818 he wrote, "Beer apparently seems to have dropped the idea of extracting the cataract by the intracapsular method." Thus Beer through his professional life evolved from performing solely intracapsular extractions to returning to extracapsular extractions.

An important contribution to cataract surgery by Beer was his triangular cataract knife (Fig. 2). Hirschberg notes that this was a refinement of Berringer's "half-moon knife" introduced in Bordeaux in 1756. With its use, Beer devised "the final classic acurate incision." The aqueous escaped slowly and the iris stayed in place without prolapsing onto the knife. In 1817 in C.F. Graefe's *Repert. augenärzt. Heilformeln* Beer describes an anterior chamber irrigator. This was composed of a water container which was elevated and

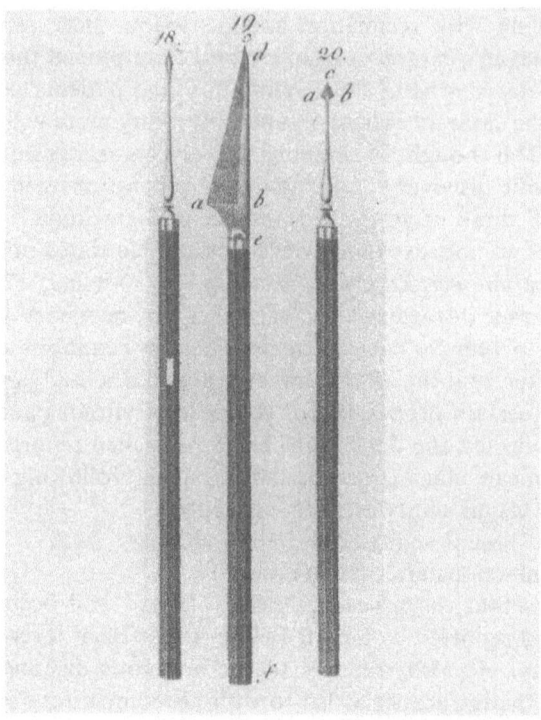

Fig. 2. The last plate in his textbook is concerned with surgical instruments and Beer presents nearly 30 of them. Many of the instruments are of his own design.

We are reproducing here the three instruments mainly concerned with cataract operations. On these three instruments alone Beer wrote a legend extending over more than three pages.

Number 18 is a lancet-shaped cataract needle which was used for couching. Beer emphasizes that the exact measures of this instrument have to be followed otherwise other parts of the eye could be injured.

Number 19 is Beer's own cataract knife. Beer says that it is better than the one used by his "most venerable teacher Barth." He goes on to emphasize that it is easier and safer than any other cataract knife, e.g. the one by Wenzel or the one by Richter. Again, the measurements are crucial for a safe and adequate incision. The handle is octagonal so that it can be better grasped.

Number 20 is a cataract lancet which is used to incise and open the anterior lens capsule. Beer used it not only to perform a discission, but mainly for spearing the cataract in order to perform an intracapsular cataract extraction, a method which he favored over all the others. He points out that this instrument is far superior to the old cystotome.

surrounded by ice. A tube led from the container into the eye where it turned slightly upward and ejected at its end a small fountain of fluid.

In performing a cataract operation, Beer objected to Dehais-Gendron's suggestion that the patient lie on his back after the incision had been completed. Beer desired the patient to be sitting upright throughout the procedure. He also rejected the proposal to rest the elbow of the surgeon's arm on the knee. He wrote: "it is one of the principal rules for the surgeon to keep his hands as free as possible. This rule is especially important for the cataract operation. A surgeon who is slave to his position or who cannot operate as well with the left as with the right hand should better stop operating."

Although opium, sleeping potions and various other medications had been used in past centuries to allay the pain of surgery, in Austria in Beer's day the cataract extraction was always performed without anesthesia. Classical surgeons like Beer also rejected fixation instruments because, according to Hirschberg, they did not have any good ones available. It was not until 1820 that J.D. Bloemer of Berlin devised the first useful fixation instrument.

The French priest Desmonceau made the suggestion that myopes should have their clear lenses extracted to improve their visual acuity. Beer's initial reaction to this in his *Repertorium* (1799) was to reject it out of hand. In 1817, in his *Augenkrankheiten* he considers the question in more detail and concluded, "Is it not possible to help a patient with an extremely severe myopia by extracting the lens?" The success of the cataract extraction in patients who before the cataract had a high myopia would speak for such an approach; no other patient has such a good vision after the operation than the myope. His vision improves after the cataract operation to an extent that he could not imagine. What is, however, the success rate of this operation especially when we extract a clear lens? It is possible that the myopic patient who sees quite clearly all the instruments which approach his eye becomes apprehensive and resistant. Would this not make the final result more uncertain than in a usual cataract extraction? It is not difficult to extract a lens that has not become opaque? Somebody who has never tried it, can really not evaluate it. It does, however, seem worthwhile to try this procedure at least on one eye of highly myopic patients."

Beer also became interested in visual physiology and psychology particularly in patients who were born blind and regained their vision after cataract operation. Beer had, in fact, operated on fourteen patients who were born blind and observed that it took some of them more than four weeks to tolerate intense light. He found that these patients recognized red, yellow, and blue before the operations. He stated that red was unpleasant for them but blue and green quite pleasant. He found most curious the fact that all of them "quickly and completely lost their previous admirable happy-go-lucky attitude." After surgery they recognized objects only when they also used their sense of touch. In the initial post operative period they had difficulty judging distance and also had difficulty with diplopia. Beer noted with interest that these patients never saw objects inverted.

Beer had thus carefully evaluated couching or reclination and had not rejected this entirely. He had determined the indications for discission of the lens, and he had enthusiastically endorsed and refined Daviel's extraction, contributing his valuable triangular knife and irrigator. He had determined through trial and error those cases best served by intracapsular extraction as opposed to extracapsular extraction. These experiences he had shared with his students, and through them spread his teachings and techniques throughout Austria, Germany, continental Europe, England and even America.

Of perhaps even greater importance than his contributions to cataract surgery was his invention of iridectomy. Numerous infectious diseases which plagued Europe at the time left in their wake scarred corneas and occluded pupils. Beer in 1798 demonstrated that it is possible to form an "artificial" pupil by excision of a wedge-shaped piece of iris — the first iridectomy. In 1805, he published his method in which using his triangular knife or a keratome he made a small incision at the limbus and then pulled a fold of iris out of the eye with a forceps. He excised this tissue with a pair of scissors. This procedure produced a new peripheral pupil and restored some vision to eyes with an occluded pupil or a central corneal opacity. Beer notes that he was motivated to devise his procedure because of imperfections of the procedures of Wenzel and others which were essentially iridenclyses or iridotomies. He experimented with it during an eight year period on 37 patients and in 32 of theses he had success. Beer stated, "without being proud or arrogant I would like to state that I am going to stick with this simple procedure and teach it to my students in good conscience. The procedure can be performed by even an unexperienced but skillful neophyte." Hirschberg notes, " this operation underwent all kinds of complicated modifications before the simple and natural procedure was generally accepted." It is to Beer's credit that the superb English surgeon, Benjamin Travers adopted both Beer's procedure for cataract extraction and iridectomy conforming exactly to the techniques that Beer proposed.

In the study of medical ophthalmology, Georg Joseph Beer's greatest contribution was the first precise and concise description of iritis, given in his *Augenkrankheiten* of 1813. Hirschberg tells us that in the Hipprocratic collection we find descriptions of conditions which are recognizable as sequelae of iritis, specifically irregular and constricted pupils. Further, in the Greek canon of ophthalmology, phthisis is described as a disease of the pupil which becomes "constricted, dark, and dirty." Galen also briefly mentions inflammations of the iris. Hirschberg notes that the Arabic canon of ophthalmology is more extensive than the Greek one and speaks of an "earthy, hard, occlusion of the pupil and of an abcess of the iris."

Hirschberg continues: "During the renaissance of ophthalmology in the eighteenth century, iritis is mentioned and briefly described by Maitre Jan and by St. Yves." The textbook by Dehais-Gendron mentions the inflammation of the uvea and an abcess. The textbook by Plenck speaks of an inflammatory miosis which originates from an iritis or uveitis. Plenck adds that it originates from hyperemia of the white coat, the iris becomes red and the pupil constricted so that the patient sees less. There is photophobia, pain, and an intolerable pulsation in the head and in the eye. Richter also describes the "Phlegmone oculi" or internal inflammation of the eye.

In Beer's first text book of 1792, he gave a good description of iritis under the rubric "syphilitic iritis." This was, in fact, the first precise description of syphilitic iritis ever written. In his later textbook in 1815, Georg Joseph Beer presented an even more comprehensive description of iritis. With regard to syphilitic iritis he proposed for the first time the systemic application of mercury. His observations were confirmed and elaborated upon by Saunders (1806), Travers (1816, 1818) and von Ammon (1835, 1839, and 1843). Beer made the observation that a "gouty inflammation" is difficult to diagnose when the first attack of "gout" affects the eye directly. The "rheumatic" ocular inflammation can be similar to the "gouty" one and both of these may take the form of an iritis.

Although Beer offered the clearest concept of iritis to that time, his assignment of inflammation to other tissues of the eye was vague. This is understandable in view of the lack of the ophthalmoloscope or slit-lamp, and the absence of good histopathologic correlation in those years. Beer confined himself to the term "ophthalmia," subdividing it into "ophthalmia externa" and "ophthalmia interna" and occasionally using the term "blephar-ophthalmia." Hirschberg finds this term more "correct" than either ophthalmitis or panophthalmitis. The legion of diseases of the eye ending in -itis were enumerated in subsequent years. Most of these are to be found in the work of Anton Rosas, Beer's student and eventual successor as professor, who in 1830 completed the list with blepharitis, conjunctivitis, keratitis, keratoiritis, sclerotitis, chorioditis, retinitis, hyalitis, and both phakoideitis and lentitis.

A significant defect in Beer's *Lehre der Augenkrankheiten* published in 1792 was his failure to recognize trachoma. Hirschberg notes that Table 1, Figure 4 in this work is an illustration of trachoma. On the basis of this figure, Otto Becker deduced that trachoma occurred in Europe even before Napoleon's campaign in Egypt. Hirschberg adds: "This should have been well known to everybody." Beer had neither in 1792 nor in 1799 a correct concept of the disease which the Greek authors had already called trachoma. This can be seen clearly in his *Repertorium* (II; page 24). His student von Walter recognized and mentioned this in 1821: "If the venerable Beer had seen several such patients, he would not believe that this (contagious Egyptian) ophthalmia is a simple inflammation of the glands of the lids and that the poor results are only the effect of the poor treatment given by the Egyptian, French and English physicians."

Beer also did not have a good grasp of gonorrhal inflammations of the eye. Hirschberg notes that Samuel Theodor Quelmalz (1696–1758) who served from 1737 to 1757 as professor of anatomy, physiology, surgery, pathology and therapy at Leipizg, pointed out 100 years before Semmelweiss the frequency and importance of ophthalmia neonatorum and stated that the cause is the purulent vaginal secretion in the mother and is therefore the result of gonorrhea in the father. William Rowley (1743–1806) in *A Treatise on One Hundred and Eighteen Principal Diseases of the Eye and Eyelids* (London: 1790) states, "We know that this kind of ophthalmia is transmitted by the incidental touching of the eye with a finger that had before come into contact with a venereal exudation." Although Hirschberg finds this important statement repeated in the writings of Astruc and van Swieten it was apparently ignored by Beer. Beer did ridicule Rowley's treatment for this disease which included blood letting, antiphlogistic medications, and oral sublimate. Beer contended that ophthalmia neonatorum was caused by polluted air, especially in the lying-in hospitals and in orphanages, the carelessness with which newborn are exposed to all kinds of light, the rough washing of the eyes of the newborn with a coarse soap, and the pouring of cold water during baptising onto the perspiring head of the newborn. Furthermore he stated that when gonorrheal blenorrhea resulted from direct infection, it was usually mild, while when resulting from metastasis it was severe.

In the treatment of ophthalmia, Beer's armamentarium consisted of cold compresses and topical blood letting by leeches and scarification. Two curious medications which were popular at the time and received Beer's endorsement were the fat of vipers and millipedes. Hirschberg traces the use of the fat of vipers in eye ointments to Galen, Aetius, and Ibn Sina. Its resurgence in popularity he attributes to Hans Sloane, founder of the British Museum and second president of the Royal Society. Sloane in 1745 wrote a monograph entitled *On Sore Eyes* which promoted an ointment consisting of the fat of vipers, zinc oxide, iron oxide, and aloe. The use of millipedes baked in a soap found popularity following the report of the cure of Hussar, blind from typhus, by the Prussian army surgeon Johann Leberecht Schmucker who used this medication.

Although Beer had a faulty grasp of ophthalmia neonatorum, he was a pioneer in the field of ocular hygiene. In addition to the cold compresses previously mentioned, he advocated submersion of the eyes with the lids open in cold water. As discussed below, he wrote an important book for the layman on ocular hygiene and care of the eyes.

A cause of foreign body inflammation which Hirschberg considered significant was the introduction of "husks from bird feed" which dropped into the eye. Hirschberg traces recognition of this malady to Beer's description of "half a husk of a hemp thrown into the eye by birds" in his *Augenkrankheiten* of 1813.

Hirschberg regards Beer's discussion on glaucoma as "one of the best which up to then appeared in the literature." Beer shared Demours' view that glaucoma, next to cancer, was the most malignant disease which could afflict the eye. Glaucoma was considered relentless and incurable. "Hydrophthalmia," defined as an extension of all the coats of the eye, especially of the anterior segment, was considered less hopeless. The etiology was believed to be a constriction or occlusion of the excretory vessels with a normal or increased function of the afferent vessels and the treatment was evacuation of the aqueous. Beer in his *Repertorium* stated, "In paracentesis we perform a perforation with a lancet, needle, or trochar through the sclera or the cornea . . . The main indication for paracentesis is hydrophthalmos." Beer stated that he always opened the cornea with a cataract knife, even if it was the vitreous which was mainly enlarged. Beer, however, was discouraged by the meager results of this attempt at a cure.

In his *Augenkrankheiten* of 1817, Beer gave one of the best descriptions of constrictions of the visual fields to that time. In this work he attempted to differentiate circumscribed visual field defects ("visus interruptus") from floaters ("visus muscarum"). Beer believed that floaters were a beginning sign of gutta serena and Hirschberg applauds his astute observation that they can be the first symptom of a retinal detachment (made nearly half a century before the ophthalmoscope had been invented.) Beer unfortunately used the terms "scotoma" to describe floaters and it was left for Sichel and von Graefe to properly define this term.

Beer made important contributions to the understanding of both congenital and senile changes in the eye. In his 1813 monograph *Das Auge*, he illustrated coloboma of the iris. In his 1817 *Augenkrankheiten*, he beautifully described the arcus senilis which he referred to as "Marasums senilis corneae." He attributed this to an occlusion of the small vessels at the limbus similar to vascular sclerosis in older patients. Hirschberg notes that Greeff repeated this assumption in his 1906 text.

An area in which Georg Joseph Beer was far ahead of his time was with regard to refractive errors. Hirschberg speculates that this resulted from his knowledge of the work of the mathematician George Albert Hamberger who published in 1696 a book entitled *Optica Oculorum Vitia*. Hirschberg states, "This is the first monograph on refractive errors — the root, so to speak, from which 170 years later the classical book by Donders evolved." Yet another area in which Beer had an understanding superior to that of his peers was with regard to lid abscesses and orbital cellulitis. While Schmidt and others attributed these symptoms to lacrimal gland inflammation, Beer more clearly understood their pathogenesis.

Georg Joseph Beer's contributions

The only complete bibliography and discussion of the writings of Georg Joseph Beer is that by Hirschberg. The following is a summary of Hirschberg's exhaustive discussion together with some of the present author's observations. A hallmark of Beer's books are the extraordinarily fine illustrations, attesting to Beer's artistic talent. These retain their clinical interest to this day. His illustrations of instruments are of historical importance in allowing the modern reader to identify the various knives, scissors and forceps used in Vienna in the late eighteeth and early nineteenth centuries. Beer's books are considered in chronological order.

Praktische Bemerkungen über verschiedene, vorzüglich aber über jene Augenkrankheiten, welche aus allgmeinen Krankheiten des Körpers entspringen (Practical comments about various eye diseases, especially, however those which are derived from systemic diseases). Vienna: 1791.

This is the first monograph ever published dealing with ocular signs of systemic disease. It deals with lacrimal fistulas, trichiasis, adhesions of the lids, lid ulcers, epiphora, and ocular inflammations. He illustrates through anecdotal cases the ocular changes caused by small pox, measles, venereal afflictions, gouty and rheumatic diseases, scrofular, and dietary deficiencies.

Praktische Beobachtungen über den grauen Star und die Krankheiten der Hornhaut (Practical observations on the cataract and corneal diseases). Vienna: 1791.

This is a comprehensive and accurate description of cataract and its operation as well as a consideration of corneal diseases including pterygium, corneal scars and staphyloma.

Lehre der Augenkrankheiten (The knowledge of eye diseases). Vienna: 1792.

Although this work bears the same title as the 1813–1817 text, it is, in fact an unrelated book and should not be considered a first edition of the later work. Its major strength is in the several personal observations Beer makes. Beer attempted to include an "index latino-graecus et gallicus" of ocular diseases, but according to Hirschberg this contains many errors. Hirschberg also notes that "quite a few paragraphs in the . . . book are taken from other publications, especially from Richter." The drawings are crudely done in comparison to Beer's later work. Beer significantly makes no mention of this book in his 1813–1817 *Augenkrankheiten*.

Bibliotheca ophthalmica . . . Repertorium aller bis zu dem Ende des Jahres 1797 erschienenen Schriften über die Augenkrankheiten (Complete ophthalmic repertory of all publications on ophthalmology up to the end of 1797). Vienna 1797.

Hirschberg uses this reference extensively in his definitive history, although he complains about its numerous grammatical and historical mistakes. He recognizes this to be "a work of remarkable diligence and . . . the only one of its kind" and concludes, " We have to excuse Beer (for his mistakes) in these respects. Somebody who makes history does not always have the facility to write it. Not everybody is Gaius Julius Caeser." This is a tremendous resource for the ophthalmic historian fortunate enough to have a copy. If an alphabetical index is someday appended it will be even more useful.

Methode, den grauen Star mit der Kapsel auszuziehen, nebst einigen anderen Verbesserungen der Star-Operation überhaupt (A method to extract the cataract within the capsule with a few comments on improving the cataract operation). Vienna: 1799.

An important exposition of Beer's method of intracapsular extraction, this book remains of interest to the modern day surgeon.

Auswahl aus dem Tagebuch eines praktischen Augenarztes (Selections from the diary of a practicing ophthalmolgist). Vienna: 1800.

Beer states: "It had always been the purpose of my publications and lectures to propogate the study of eye diseases. — A few have criticized me (nobody can please everybody), but I continued in my endeavor. . . . The thoughts enforced my intention to continue with my clinical lectures which

I have begun again during the last year; I shall begin these lectures with a printed program. . . ." This is a precise description of gonorrheal ophthalmia which, on the basis of 100 cases, Beer is convinced cannot be distinguished from ophthalmia neonaturum. Beer also describes syphilitic ophthalmia and advocates the use of topical mercury for this and other eye diseases.

Praktische Bemerkung über Augenkrankheiten (Practical comment about some eye diseases). Vienna: 1800.

Here Beer advocates Conradi's eye solution (sublimate 0.05 to 180) against catarrh as well as ophthalmia neonatorum. Chapters on dermoids and staphyloma are included.

Pflege gesunder und geschwächter Augen nebst einer Vorschrift, wie man sich bei plötzlichen Zufällen an den Augen, welche nicht eigentliche medizinische Kenntnisse fordern, selbst helfen kann (The care of healthy and weak eyes with a guideline on how to treat sudden ocular complications which do not need specific medical knowledge). Vienna: 1800. (Also Leipzig: Weidmann Bookstore, 1800).

This book is the first reasonably complete treatise on ocular hygiene. Written primarily for the layman, it enjoyed wide popularity and was translated into French and English where it underwent many editions. It contained many common sense recommendations as well as obsolete concepts. Beer warned about exposure to bright light, the need for proper artificial light, and avoidance of exposure to noxious fumes. He gave a good description of asthenopia, advising rest and irrigation of the eyes.

Ansicht von der staphylomatoesen Metamorphose des Auges und der künstlichen Pupillen-Bildung (Concepts about the staphylomatous metamorphosis of the eye and the new formation of a pupil). Vienna: 1805.

In the first part of this monograph, Beer offers an astute presentation regarding staphylomas. The second, more important, part describes Beer's operation to form a new pupil. He points out the advantages of iridectomy over the previously popular iridodialysis. He included a discussion of anatomical studies demonstrating the relationship of the lens to the ciliary processes. Hirschberg concludes, "this publication is characterized by an unusual clarity and precision."

Queries proposed to those medical gentlemen who have opportunities of observing the epidemical ophthalmia, which has long prevailed in the British

Army. Vienna: 1806. Reprinted in the Medical and Phys. Journal of London (XIV, 317–20), 1810.

This article consists of 26 questions concerning the "epidemical ophthalmia" or trachoma. Hirschberg states: "This attempt proves Beer's active investigational drive. What he himself could not possibly observe he wanted to learn from others. Whether Beer ever received a response to these questions is unknown.

Geschichte der Augenkunde überhaupt und der Augenheilkunde insbesondere (History of our knowledge about the eye and of ophthalmology). Vienna: 1813.

This work is the inaugural oration given on April 28, 1812, on the occasion of the opening of the first clinical course in ophthalmology and published at the request of Beer's students. Beer used the writings of Haller and Sprengel as his main sources. Beer carried his history to the year 1812.

Übersicht aller Vorfälle in dem öffentlichen klinischen Institute der k.k. Universität zu Wien (Survey of all events in the public clinical institute of the Imperial Royal University of Vienna). Vienna: 1813–1816.

This documents patient care and departmental affairs during this three year period. A library was started and student activities recorded. One is impressed with the favorable results of Beer's surgery.

Das Auge, oder Versuch, das edelste Geschenk der Schöpfung vor den höchst verderblichen Einflüssen unsres Zeitalters zu sichern (The eye, or an attempt to protect the most valuable gift of creation against the most deleterious influences of our age.) Vienna: 1813.

An unusual and fascinating random collection of observations and theories which give insight into Beer's personality and beliefs. This includes observations regarding patients born blind who had their vision restored by cataract observation; observations on the psychological aspects of blind patients; an anecdote on the negotiation of surgical fees; a discussion of congenital defects presumably caused by severe eye inflammations in utero; observations on the care of the eyes from birth until puberty; support for vaccination against smallpox; and condemnation of wearing spectacles for reason of fashion (Fig. 3a and b). Hirschberg notes that Beer himself had excellent eyes and could see from the suburb St. Veit the dial of the clock on St. Stephan's cathedral.

Lehre der Augenkrankheiten Volume I, Vienna: 1813; Volume II, Vienna: 1817.

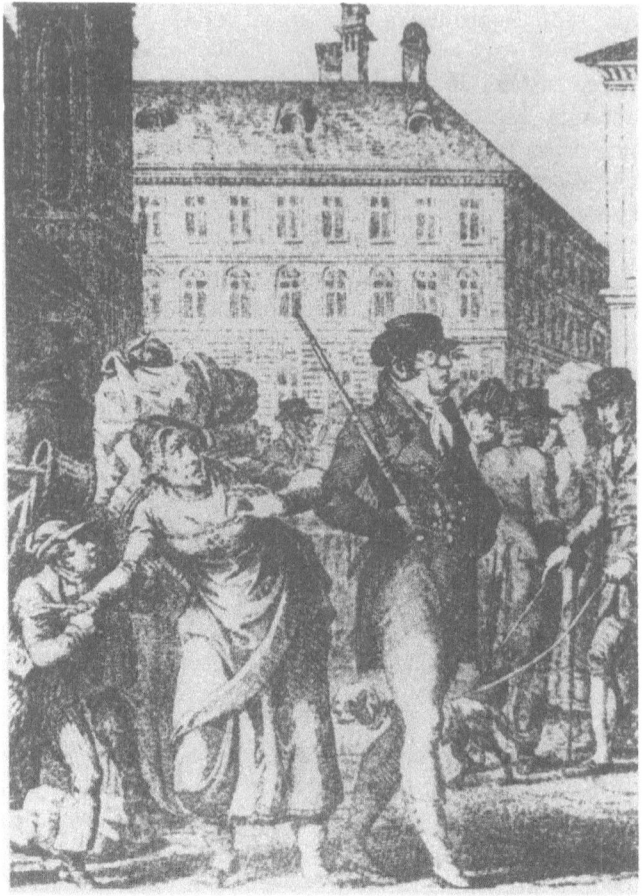

Figs. 3a and b. Illustrations from Beer's book on ocular hygiene ridiculing the wearing of glasses as foppish affectations and aberrations of the fashion.

This is the text which accompanies these notes in its edited English translation. This is considered Georg Joseph Beer's most important work and the one which Hirschberg recognizes as contributing most to Beer's fame. Hirschberg devoted 21 pages of discussion to this work, and his evaluation of this book is as follows: "We have here the product of the first professor of ophthalmology in which he presents his specialty of medicine on the basis of his 30 years of experience both in practice and in teaching. He is always cognisant of the close connection between ophthalmology and general medicine and surgery. He is a true practicing ophthalmologist, not

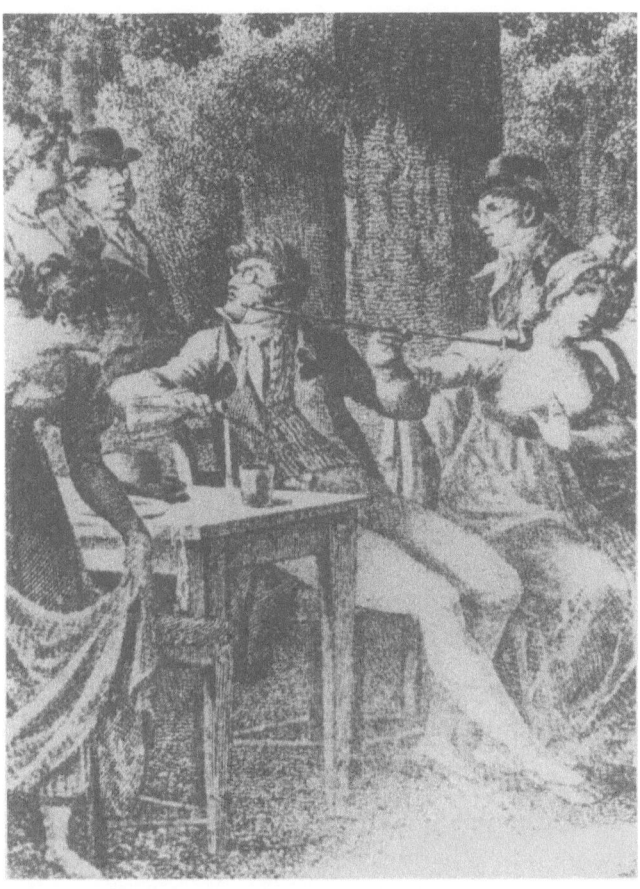

Fig. 3b.

only a cataract surgeon; he is a master of the healing arts in the real sense
of the word. He usually emphasizes the etiologic point of view and contrasts
it with the nosologic description. . . ."

The high points of the book are Beer's discussions of ocular inflammation,
and his presentation for the first time of the general principles of treating
post-traumatic inflammations. These include penetrating and perforating
injuries as well as injuries to the orbit. Beer introduces for the first time the
use of the loupe in the examination of the living eye. Hirschberg notes that
Beer's descriptions and classifications of ocular inflammation are a definite
advance and much more precise than anything to be found previously,
including the descriptions by St. Yves, Heister, and A.G. Richter. His
suggestions for treatment, on the other hand, show large gaps. The sequelae

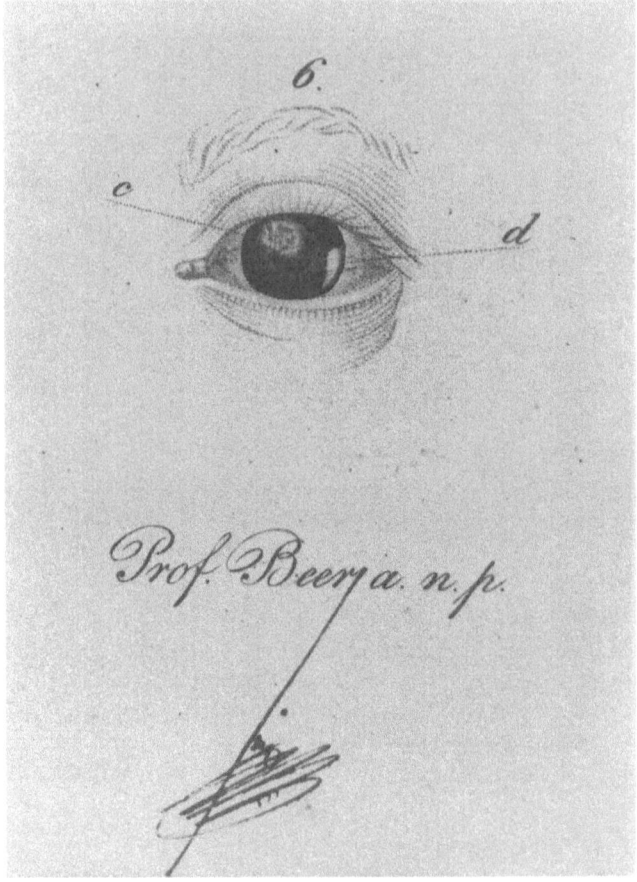

Fig. 4. This figure is from the second volume of Beer's Textbook of Ophthalmology which appeared in Vienna in 1817.

The illustrations were drawn by Beer himself. The reproductions are copper etchings and were hand painted by the author. Each plate bears in the right lower corner the signature of Professor Beer as an indication that he had painted the illustration himself.

Beer provided long and extensive legends to his pictures. He says about this figure: "We see here two grades of corneal scars which I call leukoma, painted after nature; with the letter c I have designated a chalky-white scar (albugo, paralampsis) which is due to a protein and fibrin material transformed into a pseudomembrane; — the letter d, on the other hand, shows a true pearl scar (margarita, perla) which smoothly protrudes over the corneal surface like a cut pearl. In this case the coagulated protein and fibrin material accumulate beneath the epithelium of the cornea or among the most anterior corneal lamellae. It occurs in considerable quantity and forms a true pseudomembrane."

Beer shows on this plate four different types of corneal scars all drawn from different patients. He combined two corneal scars in one picture only to save space.

of ocular inflammations are treated in detail (Fig. 4). His discussion of cataract and its treatment remains fascinating to the present day physician. Hirschberg concludes "There is no doubt that no other book on ophthalmology of the eighteenth century comes even close to Beer's contributions. Beer's books are outstanding in their content and form, are based on personal experience and keen observation, present new information and give excellent guidelines for therapy. The form of presentation is perfect. . . ."

References

Anonymous. Sketches of the Medical School of Vienna. The Quarterly Journal of Foreign Medicine and Surgery. London. Volume 1, 1819; pp. 34–9: 174–80.

(Becker B.). Catalog of Bernard Becker, M.D. Collection in Ophthalmology, 2nd Edition. Compiled by C. Hoolihan and M.F. Weimer. St. Louis, MO: Washington University School of Medicine Library, 1983.

Beer GJ. Lehre von den Augenkrankheiten, als Leitfaden zu Seinen Oeffentlichen Vorlesungen entworfen. Vienna: Camesina, 1813. (Volume 2; Huebner und Volke, 1817).

Beer GJ. A Manual of the Diseases of the Human Eye, C.H. Weller, Editor, G.C. Monteath, Translator. Glasgow: Read and Henderson, 1821.

Chance B. Clio Medica, Ophthalmology. New York: Hafner Publishing Co., 1962.

Frick F. A Treatise on the Diseases of the Eye; Including the Doctrines and Practice of the Most Eminent Modern Surgeons, and Particularly Those of Professor Beer. Baltimore: Fielding Lucas, Jr., 1823.

Frick F. A Treatise on the Diseases of the Eye; Including the Doctrines and Practice of the Most Eminent Modern Surgeons, and Particularly Those of Professor Beer. R. Welbank, Editor. London: J. Anderson, 1826.

Gorin G. History of Ophthalmology. Wilmington, DE: Publish or Perish, Inc., 1982.

Hirschberg J. The History of Ophthalmology, Volume III. The Renaissance of Ophthalmology in the Eighteenth Century (Part 1). F.C. Blodi, Translator. Bonn: JP Wayenborgh, 1984.

Hirschberg J. The History of Ophthalmology, Volume IV. The Renaissance of Ophthalmology in the Eighteenth Century (Part 2). F.C. Blodi, Translator. Bonn: JP Wayenborgh, 1984.

Jaeger E. Über die Behandlung des grauen Stares in der ophth. Klinik der Josephs-Academie (thesis). Vienna: 1844.

Lesky E. The Vienna Medical School of the Nineteenth Century. Baltimore, MD: The Johns Hopkins Press, 1976.

Mark HH. Our Ophthalmic Heritage: George (sic) Joseph Beer and ophthalmic training. Arch Ophthalmol 1963; 69: 131–133.

Shastid TH. History of Ophthalmology. In The American Encyclopedia and Dictionary of Ophthalmology, Volume XI. C.A. Wood, Editor. Chicago, IL: Cleveland Press, 1917; 8524–8904.

Documenta Ophthalmologica 68: 105–114 (1988)
© Kluwer Academic Publishers, Dordrecht

The first German textbook of ophthalmology "Augendienst" by G. Bartisch, 1583

WOLFGANG STRAUB

Universitäts-Augenklinik, D-3550 Marburg/Lahn, BRD

Abstract. This book contains various illustrations, portraits and an exact index, testimonials proving the author's professional successes as well as an accurate list of the qualities that should be demanded from any ophthalmologist. The anatomy of the head and eye is described according to Galen's ideas and Vesalius' book. Many remedies, prescriptions and medical treatments are discussed, partly showing the mystic influences of the Middle Ages.

Bartisch reports several diseases for the first time: Allergic reactions, sympathetic ophthalmia, hemeralopia, photoelectric keratoconjunctivitis, amaurosis due to toxemia of pregnancy. But most important is the part on surgery. A careful pre- and postoperative treatment is demanded in cases of cataract operations. Bartisch describes the removal of eyelashes to cure trichiasis, the operations of ptosis, blepharochalasis and the exenteration of the orbit.

This book was appreciated for a long time so that in 1686 a nearly identical reprint was published.

In 1983 the French Ophthalmological Society supported the facsimile printing of a medieval textbook of ophthalmology in German. It is the so-called *"Oftalmodouleia,"* which means *"Augendienst,"* written and published by George Bartisch in 1583 (Fig. 1). This 664 page Renaissance volume with its numerous woodcuts is a source of delight for those interested in medical history. Bartisch himself illustrated it. A luxury edition that the author dedicated to the Elector August of Saxony got lost during the last world war (Fig. 2). The Prince had to pay 25 florins for it.

The "Augendienst" was provided with an imperial privilege protecting it from being copied or reprinted. Bartisch himself shouldered most of the expenses of the publication. He stressed the fact that his book is not only addressed to doctors and heads of families, but also to patients.

In the title of his book Bartisch characterizes himself as George Bartisch from Königsbrück *"citizen, oculist and surgeon in the electoral old city of Dresden"* (Fig. 3). Königsbrück had been assumed to be his birthplace. As Münchow recently ascertained, it can be proven that Bartisch was born in Gräfenhain in 1535. This birthplace has a curious story. The name derives from an ancient established family, named Graefe, from whose branch 200 years later several famous oculists descended, amongst then Albrecht von Graefe.

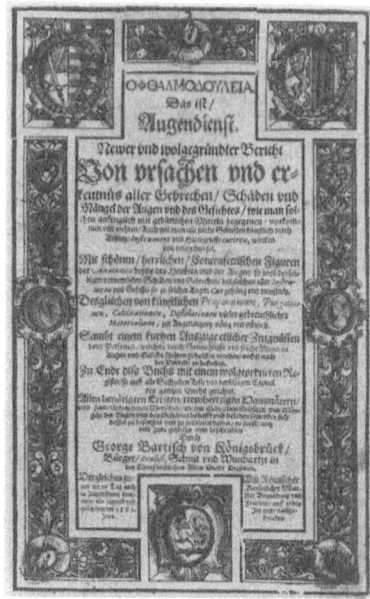

Fig. 1. Frontispiece of the "Augendienst."

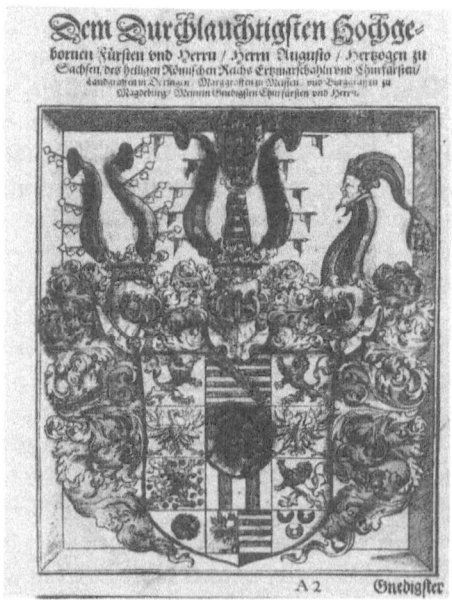

Fig. 2. Dedication to the Prince-Elector of Saxony.

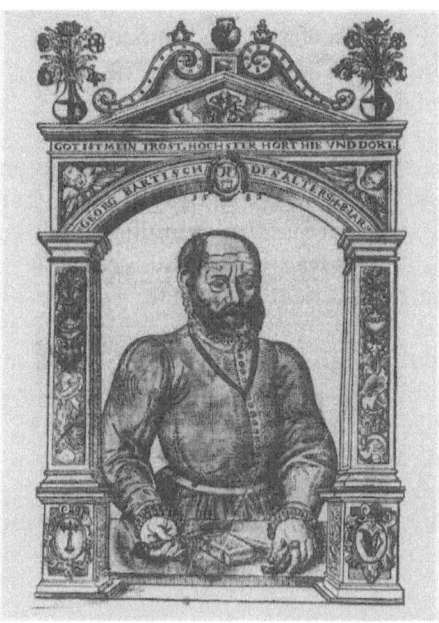

Fig. 3. Portrait of Bartisch with cataract needle in his right hand.

Bartisch was first apprenticed to a barber-surgeon. Later he aspired an education in medical science. In the preface of his book he stresses his regrets not having attended a university. He obtained his medical knowledge from practicing surgeons. According to the customs of that time he started travelling as a surgeon after having finished his training. In order to settle in Dresden and be accepted there as a citizen he had to present testimonials proving his professional successes. They fill 25 printed pages and were issued by 59 municipal councils. More than 107 excellent medical treatments are reported. From them it can be gathered that Bartisch practiced mainly in Bohemia, Silesia and Saxony, also in Prague. He became court oculist of the Elector of Saxony in 1588. Once, when a Bohemian town council requested Bartisch to operate on a blind priest, the request was rejected as without the elector's permission such a long journey was impossible.

Bartisch died supposedly in 1606.

Because of his special experiences Bartisch fought vehemently against the insufficiently trained oculists of those times.

Since to him the eye is the essential vital organ he demands the highest qualities of an eye doctor, who should not perform cataract operations in the public market place. Who does so, kills the eye. Bartisch listed 12 principles which should characterize a good oculist:

The oculist should:

1. Descend from religious honorable parents,
2. Worship God,
3. Have studied, speak Latin and know anatomy and pharmacology,
4. Be proficient in surgery and have started practicing it in youth. Persons without any appropriate preparatory training or who start their ophthalmological studies at an advanced age are incapable.
5. Have been taught by experienced oculists,
6. Have healthy eyes and normal vision,
7. Be skillful with both of his hands and able to react instantly,
8. Know how to draw in order to illustrate the instruments he needs,
9. Lead a respectable life,
10. Not be avaricious and haughty,
11. Not drink, lie and be indolent,
12. Nor promise more than he can do, and he should not praise himself.

But Bartisch admits that there are only few oculists having these attributes.

After the comprehensive introduction a discussion of the anatomy of the head and eye follows (Fig. 4). Bartisch certainly knew Vesalius' anatomy. He gives an anatomical model made of different woodcuts of the same shape laid one on top of the other so that consequently each anatomical layer and its topography became evident.

The descriptions of diseases and various remedies qualify him as an experienced eye doctor who practices as a surgeon according to the rules. He lists the traditional prescriptions and treatments for topical and systemic use. Of course, Bartisch sticks to the convictions of his time. Thus, he believes in witches and in the good or evil influences of the heavens.

Facing a bilateral massive exophthalmus displacing the eyeball beyond the lids, Bartisch doubts that this could be caused by nature (Fig. 5). He is convinced that magic is behind it. He prophylactically recommends various kinds of charms (Fig. 6), but rational remedies as well. Bartisch regards eyeglasses as injurious. To correct strabismus headcaps with fixed openings are prescribed (Fig. 7). In cases of the late onset strabismus Bartisch suggests purgatives. This medication is prepared in a pan with Bartisch's name engraved. Vesicant plasters are applied behind the ears.

We find other original disease descriptions such as occasional inflammations due to some locally applied medicines, perhaps an allergic reaction, furthermore, the sympathetic ophthalmia, hemeralopia and photoelectric keratoconjunctivitis.

The chapter about the cataract follows, differentiating various forms of it,

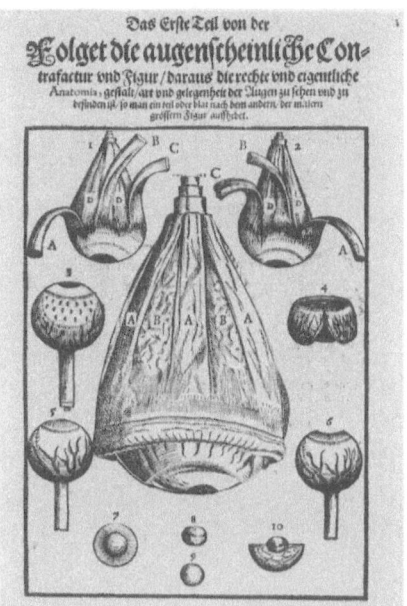

Fig. 4. Anatomy of the eye.

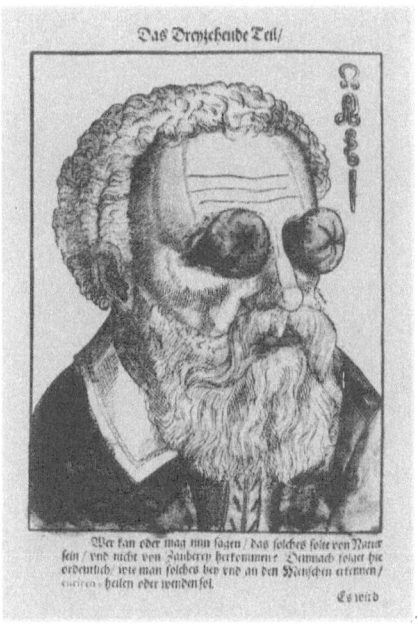

Fig. 5. Massive bilateral exophthalmus caused by magic.

110

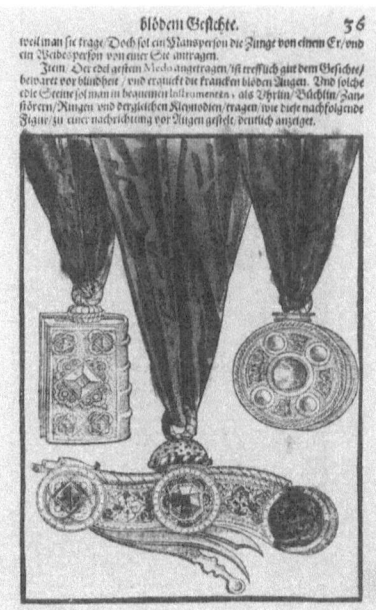

Fig. 6. Charms that should be worn on a necklace in cases of eye diseases.

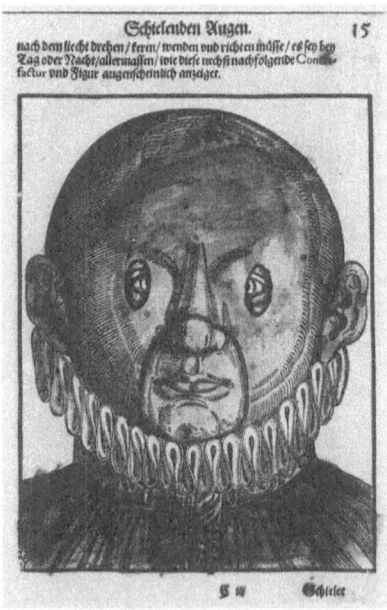

Fig. 7. Squinting mask to cure esotropia.

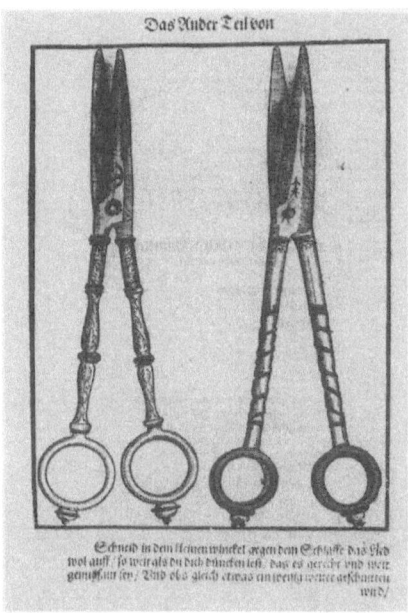

Schneid in den kleinen winckel gegen dem Schlaffe das Glid wol auff/ so weit als du dich dünckten left/ das es gerecht vnd weit genuff sen sen/ Vnd ob es gleich etwas anwenig weiter aeschnitten wird/

Fig. 8. A pair of scissors for an eye operation.

such as a green – which may mean glaucoma – white, yellow and blue one. Bartisch describes an amaurosis due to toxemia of pregnancy which disappears right after delivery.

The presentation of the artfully manufactured instruments is especially impressive (Fig. 8).

But most important is the part illustrating the surgical techniques (Fig. 9). Of course, this book did not change the traditional cataract operation, but a careful pre- and postoperative treatment is taught here: "*The needle must be perfectly clean and pure*" and it should be made out of the finest silver.

Bartisch describes new procedures to remove eyelashes for trichiasis, as well as therapy of blepharochalasis and ptosis of the lids. The latter operation is done by incarcerating the lid skin in a clip.

One of his most important novelties, however, is his orbital exenteration (Fig. 10). Hirschberg characterizes it correctly as his most original and progressive act. This operation as well as the enucleation of the globe had been unknown before him.

At first it is most important for any eye surgeon to wash his hands. The operation then is done with a special instrument which Bartisch constructed himself. It looks like a spoon with one sharp edge. After purgation and starvation on the day of the operation the patient is held by two assistants,

112

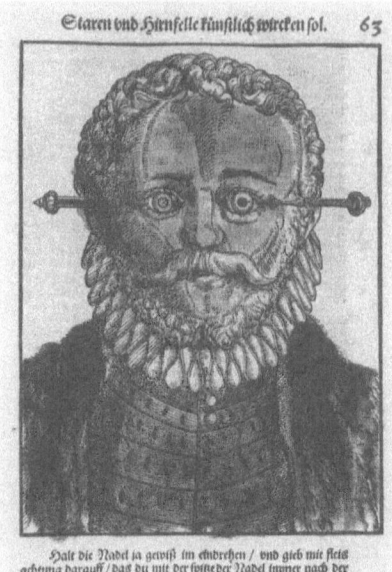

Halt die Nadel ja gewiß im ehtdrehen / vnd gieb mit fleis
achtung darauff / das du mit der spitze der Nadel immer nach der
mitte des Auges gegen der Vuea zukommest / vnd nicht etwan auff
L iij   eine seite

Fig. 9. The position of the needle during the cataract operation.

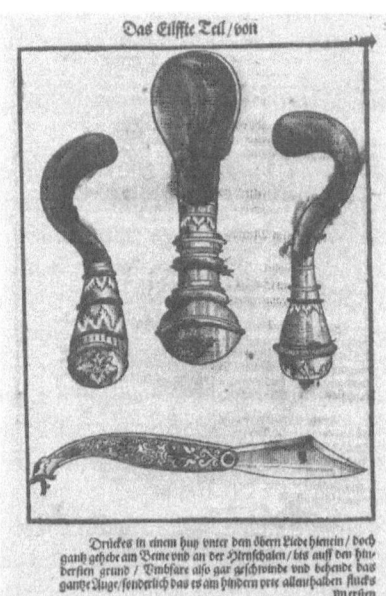

Das Eilffte Teil / von

Druckes in einem huy vnter dem öbern Liede hinein / doch
ganb gehebe am Beine vnd an der Hirnschalen / bis auff den hin
dersten grund / Vmbsare also gar geschwinde vnd behende das
gante Auge / sonderlich das es am hindern orte allenthalben sucks
m ersten

Fig. 10. Instruments for an exenteration of the orbit.

one on each side. The surgeon has to take great care of the lids in order to prevent ugly scars. The first bandage is enriched with sulfured spelter and brandy. Reading this, we cannot but admire, as did Münchow, the initiative and courage of both the surgeon and the patient.

In cases of vehement inflammations of the globe the cause of this disease – according to the ideas of Galen – should be removed. Thus, up to the middle of the 19th century a rope made out of hair helped the surgeon while removing tumors. Bartisch describes such an instrument consisting of a hot pin and horsehair, a gold wire or a wick that was stuck into a skin fold on the neck on the same side as the affected eye. The rope remained in place sometimes for months.

This treatment may produce some kind of nonspecific immunlogic reaction and might correspond quite well to what we call a stimulation therapy. It is well known from ancient times that local treatments were done by scarifications, branding irons or cupping-glasses in the area of head and neck. Perhaps this might be the reason why it has been fashionable for ladies and gentlemen to wear for ages high neck collars.

At the end of Bartisch's book is an index followed by an accurate list of "errata."

In 1584 Bartisch let somebody else publish the book. Hirschberg assumes that probably only the title page was reprinted with the following addition: "*Printed in Frankfurt am Main by Sigismundi Feyerabend, 1584.*" Otherwise, this book corresponds exactly to the one which appeared in 1583.

The real value of this book lasted for more than a century and it was the most appreciated medical compendium in those times. Who amongst us could ever expect this from any of our own publications?

In 1686 the book was reprinted in Nürnberg. The introduction points out that up to that time this book has served as a "*vademecum*" for all ophthalmologists and was then out of print. This new edition eliminated the chapters about mystic influences and magic, similarly, the prescriptions of special remedies. A better index is added. The illustrations show patients in modernized, up-to-date costumes. New is the smaller, handy size in the form of a pocket book.

Bartisch emphasized the following thesis:

Faith, honor and eyes
these three
should not be maligned.

This sentence should also be respected today.

References

1. Bartisch G. Oftalmodouleia. Das ist Augendienst. Dresden, 1583.
2. Hirschberg J. Geschichte der Augenheilkunde. Mittelalter und Neuzeit. In: Graefe-Saemisch Handbuch der Augenheilkunde, 2nd edition, Vol. 13. Leipzig: Engelmann, 1913; 332–353.*
3. Münchow W. Geschichte der Augenheilkunde. In: Velhagen, Der Augenarzt, Vol. 9. Leipzig: Thieme, 1983; 213–220.

Address for offprints: Prof. Dr. H.C. Wolfgang Straub, Direktor der Universität-Augenklinik, D-3550 Marburg/Lahn, BRD

* English translation by Frederick C. Blodi, The history of ophthalmology, Vol. 2, J.P. Wayenborgh, Publisher, Bonn (FRG).

Documenta Ophthalmologica 68: 115–120 (1988)
© Kluwer Academic Publishers, Dordrecht

The professors of ophthalmology at the University of Leipzig in the first half of the 20th century

RUDOLF SACHSENWEGER
Karl-Marx-Universität, Leipzig, DDR

History of medicine dealt principally with the curriculum vitae, the scientific and the clinical merits of the Leipzig ophthalmologists. Only little or nothing was reported concerning their personal lives. In the following, just this shall be done with the Leipzig professors of ophthalmology in the first half of our century. Their fate reflects the political and economical situation of Germany within two generations as numerously as perhaps at no other university. Four of these ophthalmologists had to suffer from the political change of the regime of the time. One of them saw the destruction of his clinic during the Second World War; two were obliged to flee from their places of work. Four lost nearly all their property. A seventy-year old ophthalmologist with a private practice in the town had nolens volens to take charge of the clinic.

In the first half of our century Leipzig had one of the greatest and most important eye hospitals in the German speaking area and always was the terminal of a professional career. During that time no Leipzig professor of ophthalmology had ever accepted another chair. The reason for this were the very favourable working conditions and the remarkably large clinic. Moreover, up to the Second World War, Saxony had many well-to-do citizens; therefore the income from private practice in the clinic was very high.

For centuries Saxony was one of the richest and perhaps happiest countries thanks to its hardworking, industrious citizens and thanks to the great mineral resources in Central Europe. Saxony has brought forth many great musicians, poets, scientists, economists, and politicians, but characteristically, no outstanding general: Since the middle of the 18th century, the Saxons lost every war or fought on the wrong side. In this way, the great kingdom of Saxony which in the 17th century reached from Thuringia to the Russian border, shrank very much, especially in consequence of Napoleon's wars. After 1945, Saxony disappeared as a state and was divided into three districts.

In ophthalmology Saxony was famous for the first ophthalmological monograph in the German language in 1583 written by Georg Bartisch the Royal Oculist in Dresden (1532–1606). This book with the title "Augendienst" or "Service to the Eyes" was published in facsimile by the French Ophthalmological Society on the occasion of its centenary. Secondly the first German full professorship of ophthalmology in Leipzig, thirdly for the foundation of the first German chair of ophthalmology in Leipzig in 1852. The Prussian universities reached this only two decades later; Albrecht von Graefe got his full professorship only in 1866.

Dresden, the capital city of the former kingdom and the later republic of Saxony, had no university. The University of Leipzig was founded in 1409 by professors and students who came from Prague because of national differences. Leipzig has one of the oldest universities in Germany.

In 1891, Professor Hubert Sattler (1844–1928) became the Director of the Leipzig University Eye Hospital. He was born in Austria and started his work in Vienna. In 1877 he came to Germany to the chair in Giessen and already in 1879 to the chair in Erlangen. In 1886 he went to Prague which at that time belonged to Austria. From there he moved to Leipzig in 1891.

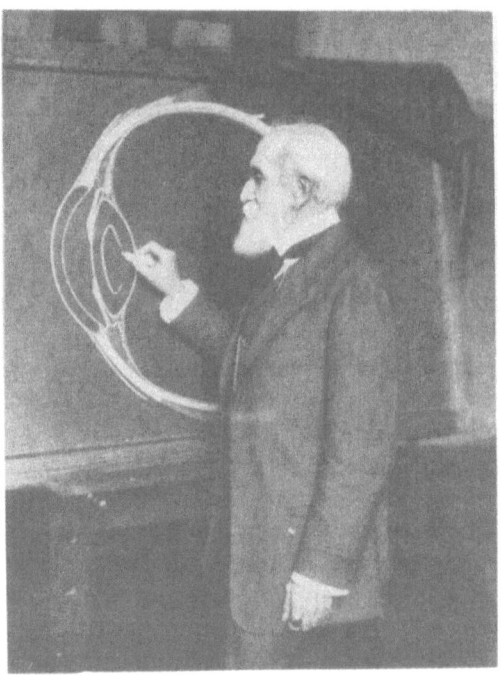

Fig. 1.

Hubert Sattler developed the Leipzig University Eye Hospital to one of the leading places of ophthalmology in Germany of his time. Six of his Leipzig coworkers got German or Austrian chairs: These were Carl von Hess in Marburg, Würzburg, and Munich; Emil Krückmann in Königsberg (nowadays Kaliningrad) and Berlin; Alfred Bielschowsky in Marburg and Breslau (nowadays Wroclaw; Bielchowsky had to emigrate to the United States in 1939 and there became director of the Dartmouth Eye Institute); Arthur Birch-Hirschfeld in Königsberg (who died in 1944 in the war); Richard Seefelder in Innsbruck and Moritz Wolfrum in Leipzig.

Sattler's main field of work was the normal and pathological anatomy of the eye and bacteriology. His excellent monograph on the Basedow-exophthalmus was published in 1910. Sattler belonged to that generation of ophthalmologists who still stood under the immediate impression of the vivid development of ophthalmology by von Graefe, Donders, Arlt and Bowman. He dedicated his life entirely to his profession, so that he entrusted the education of his only son to his parents-in-law in Tübingen. He was known as a royalist and was proud of many royal decorations.

In 1919 – after Germany and Saxony had become republics – he became emeritus – not only because of his age, but also because of his political way of thinking. Even later he was actively operated and conducted research. In 1926 when he was 83 years old, he edited his important monograph on the tumors of the eye. As a great music-lover he remained in Leipzig and regularly went to the concerts of the world famous Leipzig Gewandhaus. In 1928 he died and according to his wish, his ashes were brought to his Austrian homeland.

A second Austrian worked in Saxony, Professor Hugo Gasteiger (1899–1978). He was the director of the Eye Hospital of the new Medical Academy in Dresden, received the chair of ophthalmology at the Charité in Berlin in 1950 as the successor of Professor Löhlein who had left the GDR to accept the chair of Ophthalmology at the newly founded Free University in Berlin-West. Gasteiger also moved to the Eye Hospital of the Free University of West Berlin in 1957. After his retirement, he returned to Austria and died there in 1978.

Emil Hertel (1870–1943) the successor of Sattler, was born in Thuringia, became an assistant of Wagenmann in Jena and received the chair of ophthalmology in Strassburg. After the reincorporation of Alsace to France he was obliged to leave Strassburg in 1918 on foot, with only a suitcase. Afterwards, Hertel worked in Berlin until he received the call to Leipzig in 1920. His most important fields of research were the biology of light, optics and the construction of ophthalmological instruments. He always was in poor health and remained a bachelor up to his 72nd year. On March 3, 1942

118

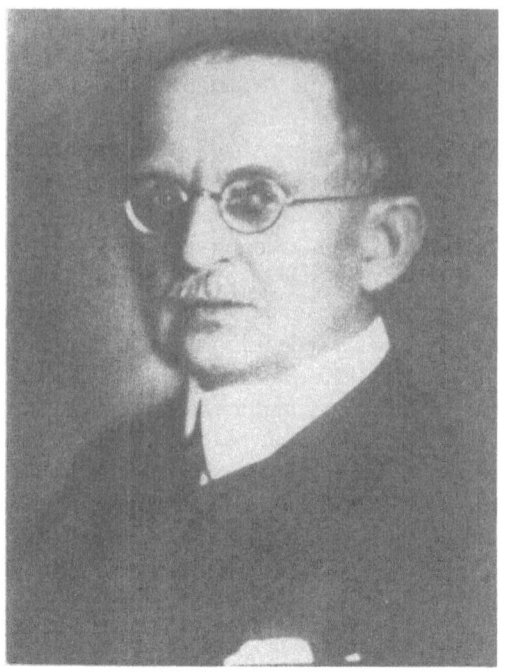

Fig. 2.

he married Johanna Schmeil. He liked fast, modern cars and travelled widely, especially to high mountains. He edited the 16th to 19th editions of pseudochromatic plates by Stilling. In 1943 he died without having experienced the destruction of his former clinic (6.4.1945) which he had modernized and enlarged remarkably. Hertel had become a very rich man, but his widow died in 1956 in Leipzig in great poverty and want, because the family's entire property was lost after the war.

During his last years in office, Hertel had to suffer very much after Hitler's coming to power, above all because he had given the vacancy of a senior physician to the Czech Dr. Kubik who later became a professor in Prague. According to the anti-Semitic laws, his assistant F.P. Fischer was dismissed in 1934. Hertel had supported this industrious and intelligent physician. Probably this had led to his early retirement in 1935 exactly when he was 65. F.P. Fischer went to Prague and later on to Utrecht; he was a half-Jew and this saved him from the worst.

The successor of Hertel became Adolf Jess, born in 1883 in Northern Germany. After working as a ship's doctor he went to von Hippel and Schieck in Göttingen and then to von Hess in Würzburg. In 1924 he received the call to Giessen and in 1935 to Leipzig. In the last year of World War II

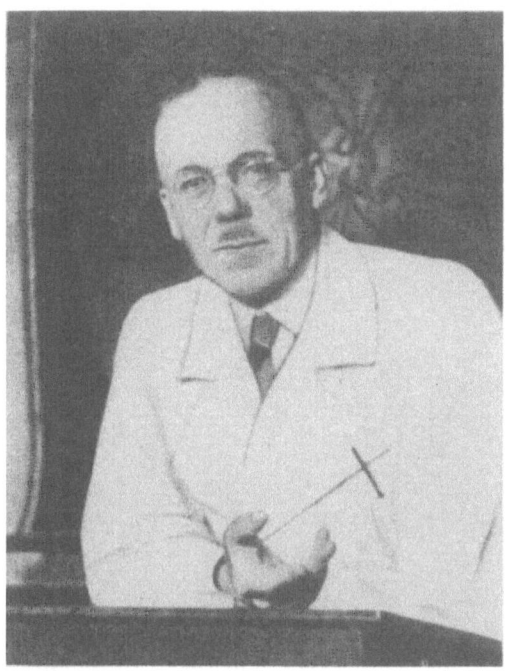

Fig. 3.

a large part of the Leipzig Eye Hospital was destroyed. This was a hard stroke of fate for him. In 1946 completely unexpectedly and suddenly he was obliged to flee directly from his clinic in his white coat to avoid a political arrest. Already in 1946 he received the call to the University Eye Clinic in Mainz in the former French occupation zone. At the age of 74 he went into retirement and died in 1977, after suffering from many diseases.

There was no successor in all the former Soviet occupation zone, because many professors had gone to the western occupation zones or had lost their positions. Therefore the seventy-year-old Moritz Wolfrum became the head of the Leipzig Eye Hospital in 1946. He was born in 1876 in Bavaria and formerly an assistant of Sattler. Wolfrum had had a private practice in Leipzig. He died in 1950. His successor became Karl Velhagen born in 1897 who had been professor of ophthalmology in Greifswald but who had lost this position in 1945. After 1945, he had a private practice in Chemnitz, nowadays called Karl-Marx-Stadt. There he was instrumental in bringing about the reconstruction of the destroyed Eye Clinic. In 1958 he went from Leipzig to the Charité Eye Clinic in Berlin, GDR.

No Leipzig professor of ophthalmology in the first half of our century could enjoy the formerly usually peaceful and prosperous life of a German

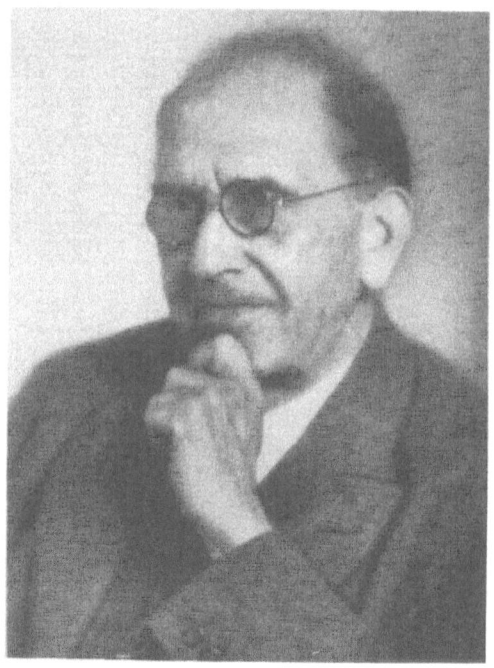

Fig. 4.

professor. Each of them had to go through many difficulties and disappoint-
ments originating in the political unrest and fundamental changes of their
epoch. In spite of it all, they mastered their fate. This seems to be no less
important than the scientific and clinical achievements for which they are
honoured.

References

Bartisch, G. Augendienst. Dresden, publ. by Stoeckel, 1583.
Sattler, H. Die Bösartigen Geschwülste des Auges. In: Klinik der bösartigen Geschwülste. I
   (P. Zweifel and E. Payr eds.) Leipzig: Hirzel, 1924.

Address for offprints: Prof. (em.) Dr. sc., Rudolf Sachsenweger, Universitäts-Augenklinik,
Liebigstr. 14, 17010 Leipzig, DDR

Documenta Ophthalmologica 68: 121–124 (1988)
© Kluwer Academic Publishers, Dordrecht

"Eye Injuries" by the Byzantine writer Aetios Amidinos

J. FRONIMOPOULOS & J. LASCARATOS
Neofytou Bamva St. 6, Athens 138, Greece

Abstract. The authors give a short report of the "Injuries of the Eye" by the Byzantine writer Aetios Amidinos.

He wrote 16 medical books, among them "The 7th Logos", including Eye Diseases. In all his writings, there is a substantial resort to ancient medical literature, mainly to the books of Galen. He describes the Eye Injuries in 5 chapters with remarkable critical ability and suitable treatment.

Thus he is acknowledged as one of the most cultured and productive writers of that period.

Aetios Amidinos, a famous physician and gifted writer of the Byzantine era, was born in Amida, a town on the banks of the Tigris, in Mesopotamia. He lived at the beginning of the 6th century A.D., studied medicine in Alexandria and was court physician to the emperor Justinian in Constantinople.

During the Middle Ages, when Athens University was transferred there, Constantinople was the richest, noblest and most beautiful of cities, celebrated as the center of culture and science.

It is due to the spiritual and intellectual people of Alexandria and the Byzantine zeal for learning, that we owe the preservation of all the great classical masterpieces and medical books of ancient Greece. But the transfer of Greek and Roman culture to Byzantine Christianity established a fixed and rather slow-developing period for medicine; under the influence of Christianity, medicine became dogmatic, guided by the principle that all medical writings ought to be held as authentic dogmas of faith and did not allow alterations of any kind.

The Christian physicians, most of whom were priests and bishops, proclaimed the importance of faith in the Nazarene and the gospels. Consequently, after the decay of Rome's idolatry and mysticism, people were passionately attached to Christianity, for the salvation of both soul and body.

The best care for the patients was entrusted to the bishops and under the church's supervision, hospitals were established in populous towns, among them Rome, Alexandria and Jerusalem, the oldest being founded in Kessaria by the bishop St. Vassilios.

Aetios Amidinos was one of the most important writers of the Byzantine period, who occupied himself with medical subjects, in particular the pathology of eye diseases. He wrote 16 books, one of which, *The Seventh Logos*, includes eye diseases. In his writings there is substantial resort to ancient medical literature, mainly to the books of Galen. Some biographers consider him as a compiler. Nevertheless, from the quality of his writings, he must be acknowledged as one who possesses critical abilities and discrimination in his choice of material. The historian Luigi Cornaro (1475–1566) regarded him as the greatest medical writer and he was highly esteemed by Renaissance physicians.

In this paper we will focus on the "Eye Injuries", in regard to the knowledge of the Byzantine physicians of this part of ophthalmology, which are included in the book Seventh Logos.

In the chapter "About Insects or Straw or Sand Blisters in the Eyes", he described with accuracy the following measures of treatment:

"On the entrance of a mosquito or other insect in the eye, you must close the other eye and open the affected one; thus the insect is automatically rejected.

When straw or sand enters the eye, you can use the same method. If this fails, you can take it out using a ring or irrigating the eye with water, milk or honey. If, after all these measures, the foreign body still remains attached to the eye, you can remove it by using one of not contaminated or not strong medicine".

In the same chapter he described "Eye injuries from splashes of lime". In these cases he advises prolonged irrigations with water and milk, in order to reduce the burning action of the lime, which can also be neutralized by egg white or rose-oil or olive oil.

In another chapter "About ulcers from burns" he points out the formation of hard coagulation necrosis over them and for that reason he recommends continuous irrigation with milk or egg white. He also advises special eye drops.

In the chapter concerning "Foreign bodies entering the eye and injuries from perforation of the eye bulb" he advises the following treatment:

"In cases where a small, pointed foreign body (scolopion) or a small pointed bone is pinned to the eyeball, it can be extracted by using a small forceps. The pulling with the forceps must be in a straight line, to avoid a part of the foreign body breaking and remaining in the eye.

When the foreign body is at the level of the surface of the eye's tissue, he advises applying pressure on both sides of this body, with the blunt tips of two probes. On the appearance of the foreign body through its entrance, it can be captured by the forceps and extracted. Afterwards, turtledoves' or doves' blood, or egg white is poured onto the injured eye.

In the case of delay on the part of the patient to seek treatment, the injury cannot be treated by surgical means but only by conservative methods such as anti-irritating irrigation and poultices, to help the rejection of the foreign body".

Aetios considers the Hyposphagma as always of traumatic origin, caused by contusion of the head or after rupture of vessels in the tissues of the eye.***

The treatment of eye injuries of this type includes phlebotomies or catharsis and pouring of turtledove's or dove's blood. He also recommends poultices on the lids with wine, rose-water, eggs and other ingredients.

When the inflammation has receded, he advises honey or Erasvistratos' liquid or aromatic eye drops. When the Hyposphagma is persistent, he advises a special medicine composed of child's urine, evaporated by exposure to the sun for some days, mixed in a copper vessel with honey. He also describes many similar medicines, such as Democritos' eye drops and others.

In another chapter he treats of "The Eye Injuries caused by Pinches". For this he recommends the pouring of blood or egg white and at first avoiding hot poultices. After the third or fourth day, anti-inflammatory poultices and mild eye drops can be used. He advises a special complicated treatment when ulcers appear.

A particular chapter is devoted to "Severe Injuries of the Eye". In case of a large wound to the eye, there is danger of the liquids of the eyeball pouring out and for that reason all precautions must be taken to avoid inflammation and fever. He recommends in the beginning phlebotomy as a help. Following this, special catharsis and the pouring of egg white in the eye must be used, as well as poultices of eggs and mild compresses of wool saturated with wine or rosewater. Continued treatment is recommended by pouring women's milk and eggs, vapor baths and poultices on the temples and the forehead, at some distance from the lids, thus making it possible to open the lids so that the tears can flow out.

When intense pain exists, the hair of the skull must be cut and cupping

***Aetios uses the term Hyposphagma probably not only for hemorrhages after injury, due to the rupture of vessels in the eye tissues, but also for those having today's term Hyphaema (blood in the anterior chamber) and maybe Haemophthalmus (blood in the posterior chamber and the vitreous).

glasses (ventouse) applied on the occipital region and the top of the skull. The food must be soft and wine avoided.

In case of rupture of the eyeball and loss of fluids, so that the bulb is wrinkled, the same treatment is applied, to prevent inflammation. When the existing inflammation has passed, he recommends baths and wine, to replace the lost fluids.

In this part of the Seventh Logos concerning severe injuries of the eye, a particular report is made on cases of Proptosis of the eyeball, due to a violent concussion of the head or a breaking of tissues and vessels around the eyeball. In some of these cases, the bulb is prolapsed forward, so that the lids cannot cover it. This happens after a fall from a great height or from a violent blow on the head. This injury is considered very dangerous and he recommends immediate phlebotomy, catharsis and the above-mentioned anti-inflammatory treatments with eye drops, cupping glasses and frequently applying the tip of a probe under the lids to avoid symblepharon.

In conclusion, we can say that Aetios, in describing "Eye Injuries" in his book the Seventh Logos, recommends a great number of complicated treatments, based mainly on Galen's works and those of other, physicians. However, we notice a systematic description of eye injuries, accurate observation of clinical findings and suitable treatment, both surgical and pharmaceutical for preventing inflammation, curing injuries and avoiding complications.

The old methods used by Aetios, due to lack of researches and novelties imposed by the dogmatic philosophy of Christianity which dominated at that time, by no means reduce the value of this distinguished physician. Thus he must be considered as one of the most cultured, efficient and productive writers of Byzantine medical literature and a notable medical personality of that era.

References

1. Aetii Amideni. in Ed. Alexander Olivieri Libri Medicinales V-VIII, Corpus Medicorum Graecorum. Berolini in Aedibus Litterarum, 1950.
2. Castigliani Ar. Medicine's History. Trans. in Greek by Papaspyrou N, 1961; 1: 251.
3. Lascaratos J. Hist. Report of the Greek Ophthal. from the Alexander period till the foundation of the first Universities. Bull Gr Ophth Soc 1981; 50: 322–342.
4. Vasiliev AA. History of the Byzantine empire. Trans. in Greek by Savramis D, Ed. Bekadi. Athens, 1954.

Address for offprints: Prof. Dr. J. Fronimopoulos, 6, Neofytou Vamva Str, 10674 Athens, Greece

Documenta Ophthalmologica 68: 125–133 (1988)

The lacrimal surgery of Petrus Camper and his contemporaries

C.E. VAN NOUHUYS
Department of Ophthalmology, Canisius-Wilhelmina Hospital, Nijmegen, the Netherlands

Key words: lacrimal duct occlusion, nasolacrimal duct obstruction, lacrimal surgery, Petrus Camper

Abstract. Lacrimal surgery went through a period of rapid development in the 18th century. This is all the more remarkable because at that time anaesthesia was still unknown.

In his ophthalmological textbook "De Oculorum Fabrica et Morbis", written in 1766, the renowned Dutch anatomist and surgeon Petrus Camper (1722–1789) presented a detailed review of the various operative procedures performed by himself and his contemporaries.

Introduction

The 18th century was a spectacular period of progress in eye surgery, highlighted by the introduction of extracapsular lens extraction by Daviël [1] in 1747. One of the first to perform and advocate the new operation in The Netherlands was the great Dutch anatomist and surgeon Petrus Camper (1722–1789)(Fig. 1).

Developments in lacrimal surgery during this period are less well-known. At the start of the 18th century the available knowledge in this respect had hardly risen above the level of the Greek physicians of classical antiquity. Early in the course of the 18th century, however, rapid progress was made in surgical techniques. The French physicians in particular contributed to the new lacrimal surgery of this period.

Petrus Camper and the lacrimal surgery of his time

Petrus Camper's interest in the eye was already apparent in his choice of subject matter for the thesis with which he concluded his medical study at Leiden University in 1746: "Dissertatio Optica de Visu" [2](an optical dissertation on vision, Fig. 2). He went on to successive professorships in medicine and surgery at Franeker, Amsterdam and Groningen [3, 4](Fig. 3).

126

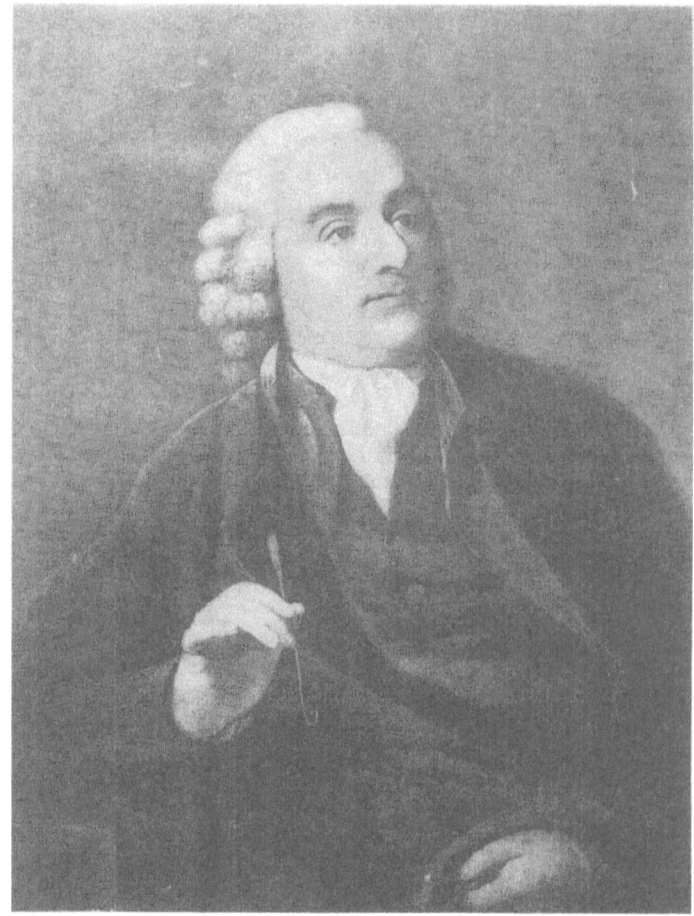

Fig. 1. Portrait of P. Camper painted by Johann Friedrich Tischbein (1750–1812) in about 1788. The portrait is property of the museum 't Coopmansûs in Franeker, Holland.

His manuscript "De Oculorum Fabrica et Morbis" was finished in 1766 but this textbook of ophthalmology, written in Latin, never appeared in print during his lifetime. The first printed edition was published in 1913, with a German translation [5].

In the first part of "De Oculorum Fabrica et Morbis" Camper presents a discourse on the anatomy of the eye and the adnexa; the second part deals with eye diseases and their treatment.

The anatomy of the human lacrimal ducts was of course well-known in the 18th century, as an illustration in Camper's manuscript demonstrates

DISSERTATIO OPTICA

DE

V   I   S   U.

QUAM,

FAVENTE DEO TER OPTIMO MAXIMO,

Ex Auctoritate Magnifici Rectoris

D. HIERONYMI DAVIDIS GAUBII,

MED. DOCT. EJUSDEM FACULTATIS, CHYMIAE ET COLLEG.
PRACT. MED. IN ACAD. LUGD. BAT.
PROFESSORIS ORDINARII,

NEC NON

Amplissimi SENATUS ACADEMICI *Consensu,*

Et *Nobilissimæ* FACULTATIS PHILOSOPHICÆ *Decreto;*

PRO GRADU DOCTORATUS, ET MAGISTERII

Summisque in PHILOSOPHIA & ARTIBUS LIBERALIBUS
Honoribus ac Privilegiis, rite ac legitime consequendis,

Publico ac solemni Examini submittit

PETRUS CAMPER, Lugd. Bat.

Ad diem 14 Octobris. 1746. ab Hora 8 ad 10. Loco solito.

LUGDUNI BATAVORUM,

TYPIS ELIAE LUZAC, Jun.

MDCCXXXXVI.

Fig. 2. Title page of Petrus Camper's dissertation.

(Fig. 4). There was doubt, however, about the mechanism by which the tears were drained to the nose. Camper considered it unlikely that a siphon mechanism was involved, as his French colleague Petit maintained. Camper thought it more plausible that the lacrimal ducts attracted the tears by capillary action.

Treatment of abscesses and fistulae of the lacrimal sac

Abscesses of the lacrimal sac were known since classical antiquity as "anchylops", while fistulae of the lacrimal sac were designated "aegylops" [6]. Celsus [7](first century A.D.) in his "de medicina" gave descriptions of the operative treatment of these conditions, which in principle boiled down to:

128

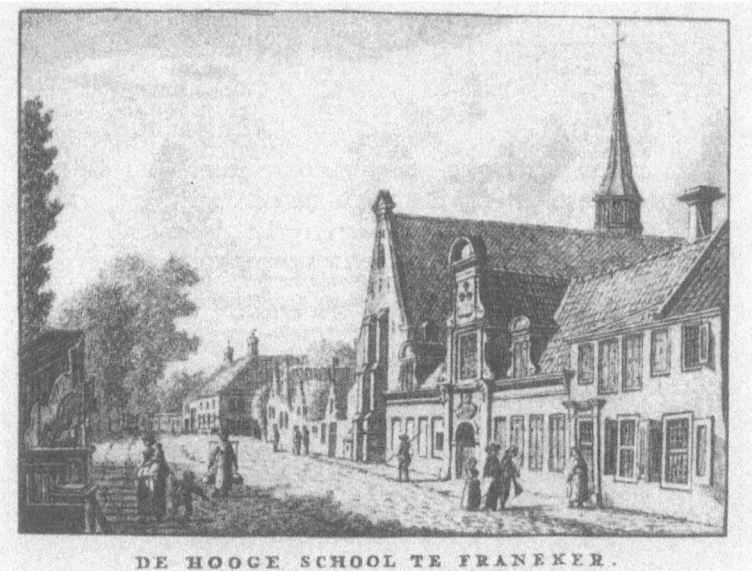

Fig. 3. The Academy in Franeker (the Netherlands) in the 18th century.

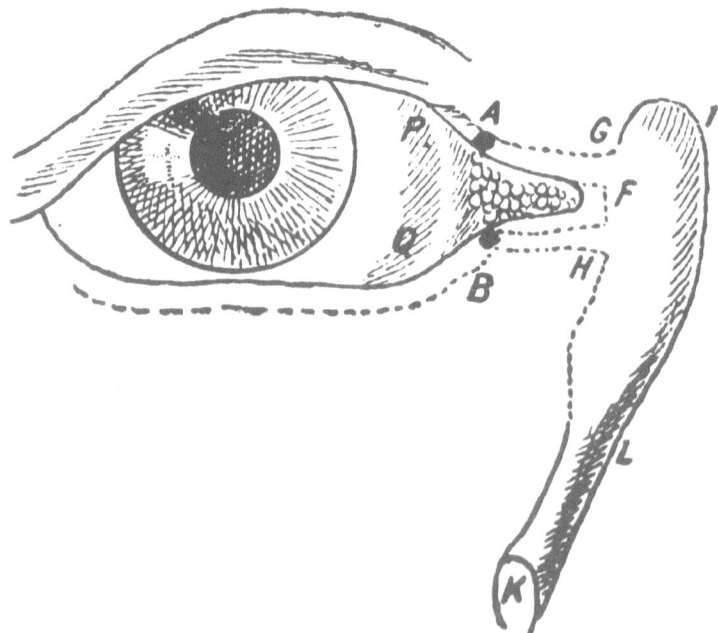

Fig. 4. Sketch of the lacrimal ducts in "De Oculorum Fabrica et Morbis".

- excision of abscess or fistula down to the bone;
- burning into the bone with a red-hot cautery iron;
- protecting the eye from damage caused by trauma or heat;
- in some cases application of corrosives (metal oxides).

The principles of this procedure were still accepted by Western surgeons at the beginning of the 18th century (Fig. 5). Camper knew the consequences of burning into the lacrimal bone from experience: in one patient the resulting skin and bone defect was so large that his speech was impeded by air escaping from the nose.

A revival of eye surgery, and no less of lacrimal surgery, started in the 18th century. St. Yves (1667–1736) [8] described in detail how a skin incision was to be made: as a crescent-shaped incision from just below the medial palpebral ligament along the orbital rim. The rough practice of burning to destroy "carious" bone was criticised by, for instance, Sharp ($\pm$ 1700–1778) [9]; he held that the lacrimal bone was best removed with a perforator. This obviously appealed to Camper, for he described how he pierced the lacrimal bone of an Amsterdam woman with a straight perforator. A few weeks after this operation the tears ran to the nose via this new route [5].

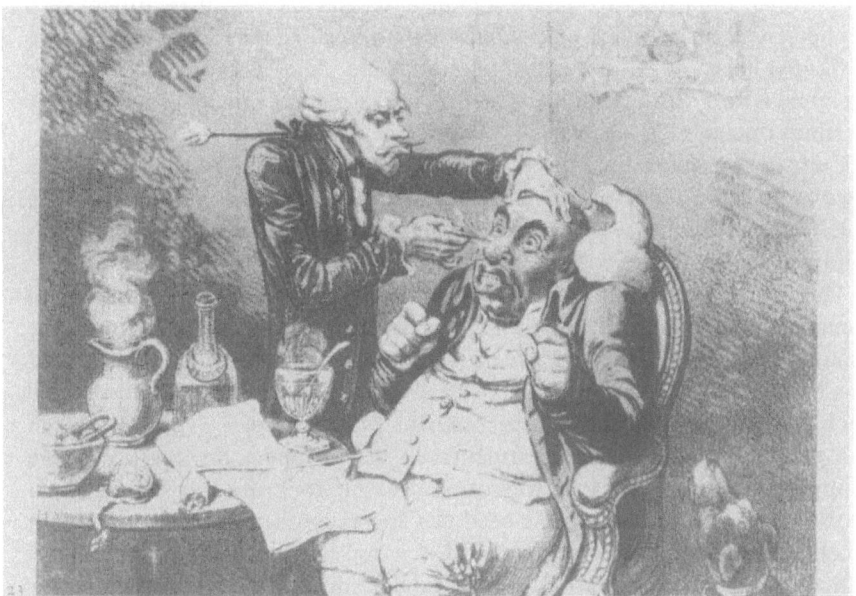

Fig. 5. Classic lacrimal surgery with the aid of the "ferrum candens" (sketched by James Gillray, 1801). From: Lyons, A.S. and Petrucelli, R.J. (eds) Medicine. An illustrated history, New York, H.N. Abrams, 1978.

It is not clear from Camper's text whether it had been his primary intention to create a new communication between lacrimal duct and nose. Evidently, however, Camper with this report was among the first to describe a primitive but apparently successful dacryocystorhinostomy.

Treatment of obstruction of the nasolacrimal duct

A condition less serious than abscess or fistula is what Camper (with Anel) described as hydrops of the lacrimal sac: dilatation of the lacrimal sac resulting from obstruction of the nasolacrimal duct. In the 18th century, surgery for obstruction of the nasolacrimal duct appears to have been a challenge to many physicians; a consequence of this interest in lacrimal surgery was the development of many new techniques, which may be summarised in three categories.

Probing of the nasolacrimal duct via the canaliculi

Anel was the first to pass a silver probe through the superior canaliculus and the nasolacrimal duct to the nose [10]. After his successful treatment of a nephew of the archbishop of Genoa in 1712 and subsequently of the duchess of Savoy, his reputation was firmly established. Anel is known also to have designed a thin cannula for introduction into the canaliculi and lavage of the lacrimal ducts (Figs. 6a, 6b).

Camper considered it a disadvantage of this new method that it was not always possible to pass the thin probe through the nasolacrimal duct: a fausse route sometimes developed, and in many cases successful probing was followed by recurrence of the obstruction.

The French physician Méjean [11] devised a method to reduce the risk of recurrent obstruction: he used Anel's probe to guide a thread through the canaliculus and then through the nasolacrimal duct to the nose. This thread was brought to view in the nose, and a slender pin was tied to it and pulled back into the nasolacrimal duct; this was repeated several times, the pin being covered with various ointments. In his comment on this procedure Camper pointed out that it was often difficult to bring the slender Anel probe to view in the nose. This need not surprise us: even in our time with excellent facilities for anaesthesia of the nasal mucosa it is sometimes difficult to reach the probe of a lacriminal duct intubation below the inferior turbinate with an instrument passed through the nostril.

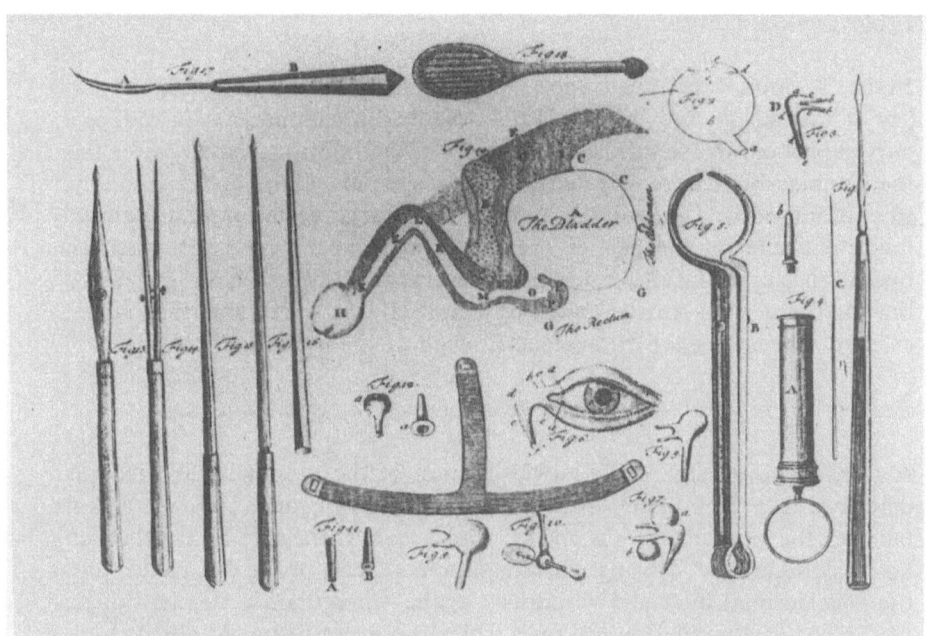

Fig. 6a. Sketch of the lacrimal ducts and instruments (right) and urological instruments (left) from the 18th century (Samuel Mihles, 1764). From. E. Bennion, Alte Medizinische Instrumente. Parkland, Stuttgart (1979) p. 144.

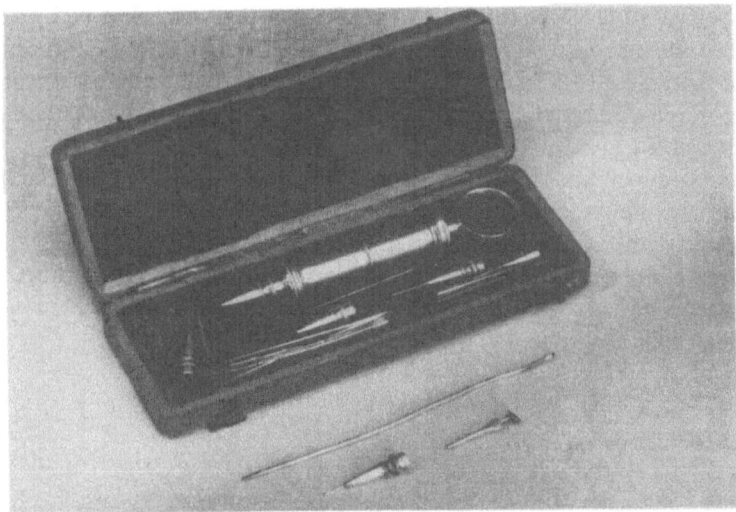

Fig. 6b. Probing set according to Anel (early 19th century). From: E. Bennion (s. Fig. 6a), 1979, p. 59.

Probing of the nasolacrimal duct via the nose.

In the "Mémoires de l'Académie Royale de Chirurgie" a French contemporary of Camper's – De la Forêt [12] – described a technique to introduce a curved probe into the nasolacrimal duct via the inferior meatus. After this the lacrimal ducts were irrigated with various fluids. Quite understandably, this technique was exceedingly difficult without anaesthesia and required much patience on the part of the surgeon. Camper's report on such an operation is brief but illustrates his perseverance: "I myself have introduced the instrument in Amsterdam, but before I was successful the patient sneezed at least a hundred times as a result of the irritation".

Probing of the nasolacrimal duct via an incision in the lacrimal sac

A third technique to relieve an obstruction of the nasolacrimal duct was described in 1734 by Petit (1674–1759), likewise in France [13]. Via a skin incision, the lacrimal sac was opened with a scalpel designed by Petit, which had a slotted blade. Through this longitudinal slot a probe was passed into the nasolacrimal duct and withdrawn again, whereupon a slender bougie was introduced and left in situ for a while to prevent recurrent obstruction. Camper gave an account of this operation, which Petite demonstrated to him in Paris in 1749. Camper's enthusiasm about the procedure was so great that he had his instrument maker make a copy of the Petit scalpel.

The revival of lacrimal surgery in the 18th century was followed by a long period of little progress in this field. Not until the end of the 19th century – more than a century later – was the technique of dacryocystorhinostomy further developed, particularly when regional and general anaesthesia became possible.

Petrus Camper was the first surgeon of his time to make a scientific study of the many new techniques and to record his knowledge (and personal experience with these methods) in an excellent textbook.

That the international reputation of this scientist was justified becomes clear when we realize that his work in ophthalmology was only a small part of his extensive surgical and anatomical studies.

References

1. Daviël J. Mémoires de L'Académie Royale de Chirurgie. Paris 1753; 2: 337–354.
2. Camper P. Dissertatio optica de visu, Leiden Netherlands 1746. Facsimile and English transl. Nieuwkoop, De Graaf, Netherlands, 1962.

3. Daniels CE. Het leven en de verdiensten van Petrus Camper. Thesis, Utrecht, Netherlands, 1880.
4. Lindeboom GA. De geschiedenis van de medische wetenschap in Nederland. Bussum:
   Fibula-Van Dishoek, 1972; 140–142.
5. Camper P. De Oculorum Fabrica et Morbis (unpublished manuscript) 1776; Library of
   Amsterdam University. German translation and original Latin text 1913. Amsterdam:
   Van Rossen, (Opuscula Selecta Neerlandicorum de arte medica, vol. 2).
6. Hirschberg J. Geschichte der Augenheilkunde. In: Graefe-Saemisch. Handbuch der
   gesamten Augenheilkunde, Vol. 14/Ch. 23. Leipzig: Engelmann, 1911; 28–43.
7. Source: J. Hirschberg: Geschichte der Augenheilkunde. In: Graefe-Saemisch. Handbuch
   der gesamten Augenheilkunde, Vol. 12, paragraph 175. Leipzig: Engelmann, 1899; 276.
8. Ch de Saint-Yves. Nouveau traité des maladies des yeux. Paris, 1722. Source: J.
   Hirschberg (see above) Vol. 14, paragraph 359, chapter 23, p. 11.
9. Sharp (undated). A treatise on the operations of surgery. Source: J. Hirschberg (see above)
   Vol. 14, chapter 23, paragraph 390, p. 124.
10. Anel D. Observation singulière sur la fistule lacrimale, Torino, 1713.
11. Méjean (year of birth and death unknown): Sur une nouvelle méthode de traiter la fistule
   lacrimale, 1750. Source: P. Camper, De Oculorum fabrica et Morbis, Part II, Chapter 2,
   paragraph 5.
12. De La Forêt. Mémoires de L'Académie de Chirurgie. Part 2, page 179. Source: P. Camper,
   De Oculorum etc. Part II, Chapter 2, Par. 4.
13. Petit JL. De la fistule lacrimale. Mémoires de L'Académie Royale des Sciences. Paris,
   1734; 135.

Address for offprints: Dr C.E. van Nouhuys, Canisius-Wilhelmina Hospital, P.O. Box 9015,
6500 GS Nijmegen, the Netherlands

Documenta Ophthalmologica 68: 135–144 (1988)
© Kluwer Academic Publishers, Dordrecht

The French Egyptian campaign and its effects on ophthalmology

MARIANNE WAGEMANS & O. PAUL VAN BIJSTERVELD
Koninklijk Nederlands Gasthuis voor Ooglijders, F.C. Dondersstraat 65, 3572 JE Utrecht, the Netherlands

Summary. Almost all soldiers of the armies involved in the Egyptian campaign fell victim to what was later called the ophthalmia militaris which we now know to be caused by Haemophilus aegyptius, N. gonorrhoea and possibly to some extent by Chlamydia trachomatis but more likely by the adenoviruses. Because of the enormous incidence of ocular infection and the controversy generated by speculation on the nature of the disease – English surgeons considered this ophthalmia to be of a contagious nature, whereas the French surgeons violently opposed this view – , the interest in diseases of the eye increased, which eventually resulted in the acceptance of ophthalmology as a separate branch of medicine.

Introduction

The French Egyptian campaign has been studied mostly for its political and military implications. Redesigned by the French Directorate as a cunning strategy to impair England's commercial interests in the Near and hopefully in the Far East and to obtain a permanent possession, it did not reach any of its objectives. Doomed from the moment Nelson destroyed the French fleet anchored at Aboukir on August 1st 1798, thus isolating the French forces in Egypt, preventing replacements of troops and so gradually eroding army size and morale, it showed Europe how strong and determined were the ambitions of the French Republic, thus hastening the formation of the second coalition.

The French military occupation of Egypt lasted less than four years, but the achievements of the French scientists that accompanied Bonaparte's army had a far-reaching effect that still lasts in our times. Every aspect of Egypt was studied including the great works of the pharaonic era and so the science of Egyptology was founded (Berthier, 1827). The discovery of the Rosetta Stone, showing a decree of a priest synod in hieroglyphs, Demotic and Greek, during the digging of an entrenchment in 1799, proved to be of infinite value as it held the key to the deciphering of the pharaonic hieroglyphs.

The Egyptian campaign also had a profound effect on the modernisation of ophthalmology. Generally speaking the standard of ophthalmology was

136

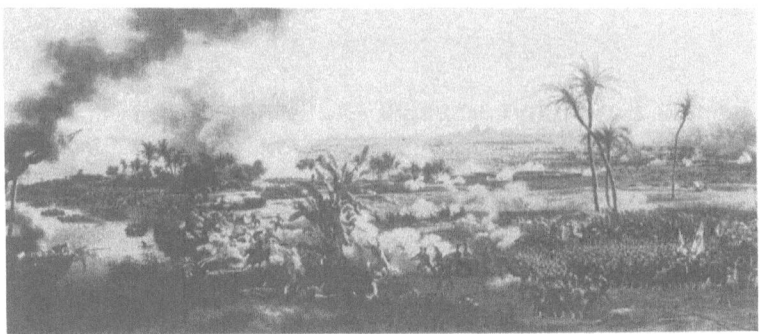

Fig. 1. The Battle of the Pyramids. On July 21st Murad Bey and his Mamelukes were decisively defeated by Bonaparte. Versailles, MV 6854. Lejeune.

low during this period and especially French surgeons and medical faculties were opposed to a recognition of ophthalmology as a speciality in medicine. Because of the great number of soldiers of the opposing armies affected with ophthalmia during the Egyptian campaign special medical measures had to be taken which resulted among others in the foundation of *Moorfields Eye Hospital* (Duke-Elder, 1965). The polemics about the nature of the Egyptian ophthalmia that raged many years even after the campaign, increased the awareness of this branch in medicine, which eventually resulted in the acceptance of ophthalmology as a speciality.

Prologue

The French Revolution has been characterized as a violent political and social change that replaced absolute monarchy by civilian republic. The French Directorate needed a permanent state of hostility in order to survive. The ruling kings of Austria, Prussia and Russia disquieted by the terrible fate of the French nobility considered this hostility a direct threat to their privileged positions and conspired to bring about the fall of the young republican state. The French army under Bonaparte, however, managed to recapture the port of Toulon from the English and because of this success Bonaparte was appointed commander in chief at the Northern Italian theatre where he managed to bring about an armistice with Austria.

The greatest menace to Bonaparte's interests was a restored monarchy which would try to make peace at once and thus dispense with his military services. The French royalists both in the National Assembly in the capital as well as in the military, moreover, were by no means eliminated in the early days of the revolution. By sending his trustworthy commander Augereau to Paris to join the Jacobin left wing, Bonaparte while still in Italy definitely

ORDRE DU JOUR DE L'ARMÉE

Lo Caire, le 30 thermidor an VI (17 août 1798).

L'armée est prévenue que, depuis le débordement du Nil, les nuits sont plus fraîches qu'elles ne l'étaient auparavant. Ce changement de l'état de l'atmosphère nécessite quelques précautions sur les vêtements. Il est indispensable d'être bien couvert pendant la nuit.

Ceux qui sont, pendant ce temps, exposés à l'air et habituellement en chemin, ou peu couverts, s'exposent à des changements dans la transpiration, ce qui peut produire plusieurs maladies et entre autres des inflammations des yeux qui, sans être dangereuses, sont fort incommodes et fort douloureuses.

Le général en chef ordonne que tout cavalier qui sera trouvé à galoper son cheval sans que sa dépêche l'y oblige soit démonté sur-le champ et le cheval remis à celui qui doit être monté après lui. Le général en chef ordonne aux officiers généraux et autres de veiller à l'exécution du présent ordre.....

Alex. BERTHIER.

Fig. 2. Ordre du jour, issued by Berthier (de la Jonquière; 1899).

managed to put down the royalist forces in what was called the coup d'état de Fructidor.

Through his successful campaigns, deft political manoeuvring and subtile propaganda Bonaparte was hailed as a national hero, much to the chagrin of the ruling members of the Directorate, who decided therefore that the popular hero had to be removed from Paris. Paradoxically, in this respect the interest of the Directorate and that of Bonaparte coincided for the fulfilment of his military and political ambitions. As the Directorate recognized England as its most inveterate enemy, not in the least because of their earlier imperial rivalries, a decision was made to threaten England's rich commerce with India by way of an invasion of Egypt. A direct invasion was not possible; the French navy being no match for Nelson's fleet.

Egypt, the land of the blind

From time immemorial the high incidence of the Egyptian ophthalmia, which reached epidemic proportions in summer and autumn, was known. Of old mainly two forms of acute inflammatory eye disorders were recognized based on the vehemence of the disease and the complications that ensued.

The acute inflammatory disease without complications was called *"ramad khafif"* and the hyperacute inflammation with serious complications *"ramad sadidi"* (Meyerhof, 1909).

The scope of this ophthalmia was brought to the attention of the European Continent for the first time by Prosper Alpinus in 1583. Later, Volney among others stressed the extraordinary high incidence of the Egyptian ophthalmia. No wonder that Tourtechot de Granger called Egypt *'the land of the blind'* (MacCallan, 1936).

But it was not until 1798, when the adventurous French Egyptian campaign started, that the full extent of this ophthalmia manifested itself to the French army surgeons. A great part of the French army of 32,000 soldiers and 1200 horsemen as well as adversaries fell victim to this disease, then well earning its name of military ophthalmia.

Bonaparte's Egyptian campaign

Bonaparte's Egyptian campaign covered the period beginning with the landing at Marabout on July 1st 1798 and ending with the rather opportunistic abandonment of his command on August 22nd 1799, leaving behind his troops that were to stay two more years before returning to France.

Bonaparte's Egyptian campaign consisted of three main periods.

— The conquest of Lower Egypt by a pincer movement, one along Aboukir Bay to Rosetta and from there upwards along the Nile towards Cairo, another pincer through the desert towards Rahmaniya by way of Damanhur. The conquest of Lower Egypt was accomplished after the decisive victory on Murad Bey on July 21st at the battle of the Pyramids (Fig. 1).
— The campaign in Upper Egypt was left to Desaix and lasted from August 25th till March 1799 when Murad Bey's Mameluke forces broke down under the strain of continuous fighting.
— The third period was the defense of Egypt against the Turkish attack, when Bonaparte marched to Syria in February 1799 to fight against the army of Damascus, which was scattered at the battle of Mount Tabor on April 16th and then double backed to Egypt in time to engage the army of Rhodes which was defeated in Lower Egypt at Aboukir on July 25th 1799.

The campaign of Lower Egypt

On the 30th of June 1798 the fleet of admiral Brueys, which transported Bonaparte and his host reached the Egyptian coast. As Nelson's fleet was

Table 1. Percent incidence of H. aegyptius (Koch-Weeks) and gonococcal infection in Alexandra (after Lakah and Khouri, 1902).

	H. aegyptius	N. gonorrhoea	Major engagements in	
			1798	1799
January	0.7 %	0.6 %	–	battle of Samhud (UE)
February	0.3	0.6	–	–
March	1.5	0.6	–	battle of Abnud (UE)
April	6.2	2.3	–	battle of Mount Tabor (Syria)
May	19.6	1.8	–	–
June	21.9	4.1	Bonaparte lands at Marabout (LE)	–
July	18.7	13.5	battle of the Pyramids (LE)	battle of Aboukir (LE)
August	14.9	33.9	battle of Salehieh (LE)	Bonaparte leaves Egypt
September	9.4	18.1	–	
October	4.0	16.4	Bilbeis, battle of El Fayoum (UE) revolt in Cairo (LE)	–
			–	–
November	2.5	8.2	–	–
December	0.3	0.0	–	–

LE = Lower Egypt
UE = Upper Egypt

chasing the French convoy on the Mediterranean, the troops were landed forthwith at Marabout that night. Bonaparte with a small army decided to march on immediately to Alexandria which was attacked by surprise and taken after a day's battle. Bonaparte ordered general Desaix's division in pursuit of the Mamelukes to forestall a co-ordinated attack of his enemies Murad and Ibrahim Bey. Two divisions followed Desaix and another was ordered to march to Rosetta to reach Cairo by way of the Nile.

By the time Rahmaniya was reached after a terribly distressing march through the desert (Richardot, 1848), the first soldiers had fallen victim to the Egyptian ophthalmia (Dupont, 1826). Initially, these inflammatory reactions of the eye were not considered dangerous but distressing and painful at the most (Fig. 2), but soon gained epidemic proportions. Present knowledge of the various micro-organisms causing inflammation of the eye shows that the period between May and August has the highest incidence of H. aegyptius infection, which explains the initial negligence (Table 1).

According to the Italian surgeon Assalini two thirds of the army suffered from the disease at the approach of autumn that year. Assalini found the majority of the inflammatory reactions to be of a relative short duration, which he estimated at 8 days on the average (Assalini, 1806), and this inflammation was well known as *"ramad khafif"*. After the decisive victory of Napoleon at the Battle of the Pyramids in which Murad Bey was defeated and Ibrahim Bey fled (Perthé, 1801), Lower Egypt could be regarded as[1] conquered, although local revolts such as in Cairo continued (Fig. 3).

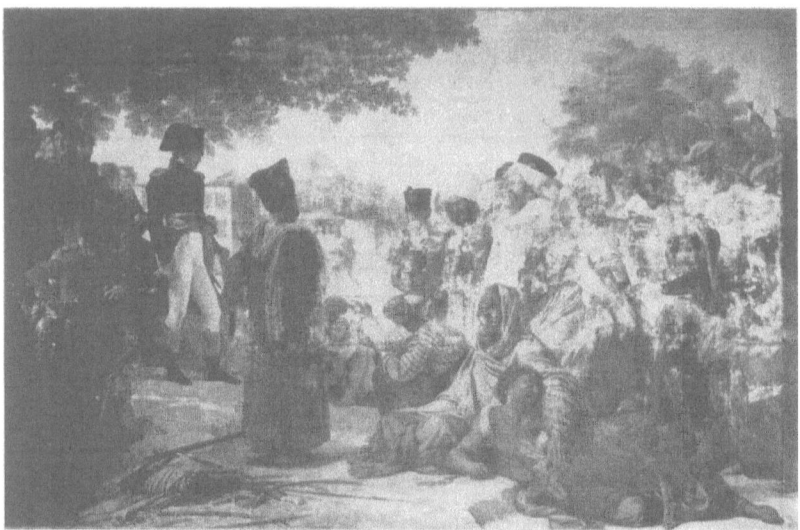

Fig. 3. Pardon of the fighters for freedom, resumption of hostilities in Cairo. Versailles, MV 1498. Guerin.

The campaign of Upper Egypt

At the end of August the campaign for Upper Egypt started. Assalini recognized already at that time that some of the ocular inflammatory reactions were of a much longer duration and of a much more serious character; these were locally known as *"ramad sadidi"*. He described this ophthalmia as a marked distension of the conjunctival vessels, massive swelling of the eyelids and pain of the eyes accompanied by a discharge similar to those observed from the urethra which Larrey (Fig. 4) interpreted as caused among others by *"l'usage immodéré des liqueuses spiritueuses et des femmes et la chaleur brulante du jour"* (Larrey, 1812).

The pacification of Upper Egypt was entrusted to general Desaix at a period in which the incidence of this blenorrhoea was at its peak. Soldiers of all ranks, including Desaix and Robin, were suffering severely from this ophthalmia (de la Jonquière, 1801). The serious ophthalmias commencing in late summer were those which we now know to be gonococcal infections (Table 1). It can be argued that although Desaix defeated Murad Bey at El Fayoum on October 7th 1798, he was not able to exploit this victory because a very large number of his soldiers was affected by the ophthalmia. The conquest of Upper Egypt was therefore extended to March of the next year (de la Jonquière, 1801).

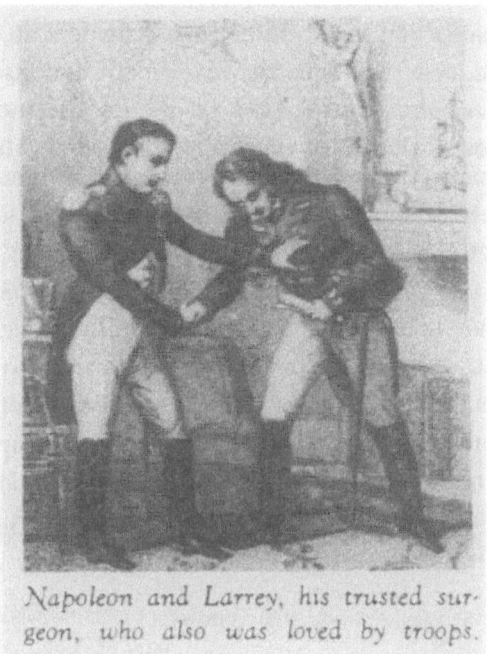

Napoleon and Larrey, his trusted surgeon, who also was loved by troops.

Fig. 4. Bonaparte and Larrey. Artist unknown.

The extent to which this infection incapacitated the fighting ability of the soldiers can be estimated from a narrative by François (François, 1903; Fig. 5). Already at the end of the year the French were forced to repatriate quite a number of blind soldiers, as well as some military surgeons. The fate of one of the repatriating groups was very tragic. One boat, carrying 150 blind soldiers and three army surgeons that had also serious ocular complications, landed on the coast of Sicily at Augusta and were mercilessly killed, while another transport that landed at Tarente had to serve in prison for a long time (Décondé, 1842).

The Turkish intervention

The declaration of war against the French by the Turks forced Bonaparte to plan a decisive offensive against Djezzar Pasha but in spite of the defeat of the army of Damascus at the battle of Mount Tabor, the Syrian campaign was carried out with limited success. Bonaparte then rapidly retreated to Egypt to meet and engage the army of Rhodes under Mustafa Pasha which he defeated at Aboukir (Fig. 6). No ocular medical records are available on the Syrian campaign nor on the period of the battle of Aboukir.

142

29 *septembre* (8 *vendémiaire*). — L'ordre du jour nous apprend que des tentatives de révolte ont lieu dans la Basse Égypte. Nous sommes nous-mêmes inquiétés la nuit et obligés de doubler les postes. Beaucoup d'hommes sont atteints d'ophtalmie et beaucoup sont devenus aveugles, d'autres couverts de petits boutons rouges ; plus de la moitié de la division est atteinte de cette maladie qui dévorait comme la gale ; un tiers au moins a mal aux yeux, et notre situation est d'autant plus critique que nous nous attendons à être attaqués au premier jour. Les positions de combat sont désignées pour les aveugles. Ils seront placés le long des murs, leurs fusils dessus et pointés à ceinture d'homme, à la distance de 30 à 40 pas. Ils ne feront feu en cas d'attaque qu'au commandement d'un chef valide, pouvant commander en temps utile. Les autres malades doivent faire les sorties avec les hommes bien portants.

Fig. 5. Narrative of Sergeant François of an episode of the battle of Salehieh (François).

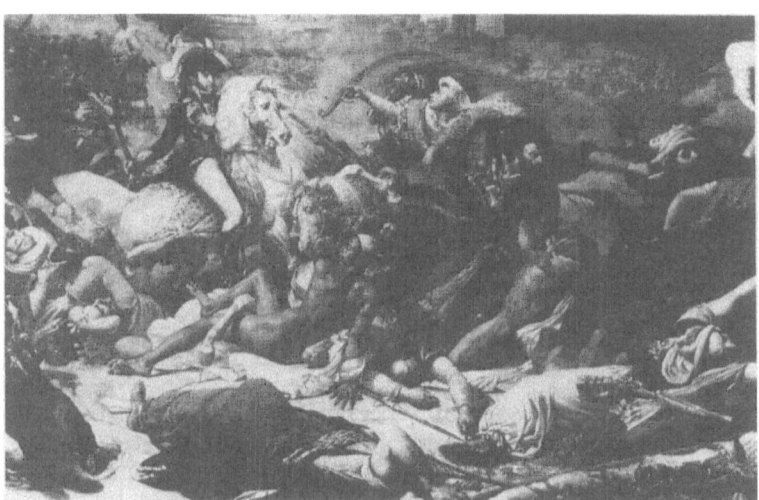

Fig. 6. The Turkish army of Rhodes was met by Bonaparte and defeated at Aboukir. Versailles, MV 2276. Gros.

Discussion

The surgeons – both French and English – attached to the armies in the Egyptian campaign were general surgeons, none of them trained in ophthalmology (Onfray, 1957). Therefore, the descriptions of what was later called *"ophthalmia militaris seu Aegyptiaca"* were not better than those already known as *"ramad khafif"* and *"ramad sadidi"*. Also, it has to be remembered that the etiology of various forms of conjunctivitis was not recognized until after the second half of the 19th century.

Not until Robert Koch had demonstrated the presence of gonococci and a small slender rod in the exudate of the Egyptian ophthalmia, later referred to as the *"Koch-Weeks"* bacillus (Haemophilus aegyptius) (Koch, 1883 and Weeks, 1886), was retrospective speculation on the nature of ophthalmia militaris possible. The importance of Chlamydia trachomatis in this ophthalmia is debatable. Although some military medical historians identify ophthalmia militaris almost exclusively with trachoma (van der Giessen, 1934), it is not likely that most *"granulomatous"* infections were caused by Chlamydia trachomatis; on the contrary, the majority of these follicular infections during the Egyptian campaign and those that ravaged the armies during the Napoleonic wars in Europe was most likely caused by what we now know to be the adenoviruses, first isolated by Rowe et al. in 1953 (Rowe et al., 1953). This view is supported by the fact that many of the corneal opacities associated with the Egyptian ophthalmia disappeared eventually (Assalini, 1806).

References

Assalini P. Observations on the disease called the plague, the dysentery, the ophthalmy of Egypt. Translated by Adam Neale. Swords: New York, 1806.

Berthier, maréchal. Mémoires du maréchal Berthier sur les campagnes des Français en Egypte. Premier partie. Baudouin: Paris, 1827.

Décondé. Histoire de l'ophthalmie dans les armées Françaises. Annales Ocul 1842; T 8: 61–69.

Duke-Elder S. System of Ophthalmology. Vol VIII, part I. Kimpton: London, 1965.

Dupont A (editor) Histoire militaire des Français par campagnes de Napoléon. Dupont A: Paris, 1826.

François. Journal du capitaine François (dit le dromedaire d'Egypte). Grolleau: Paris, 1903.

Giessen van der H. Bijdrage tot de kennis van de ophthalmia militaris of trachoom. Thesis. Utrecht, 1939.

Jonquière de la C. L'expédition d'Egypte 1798–1801. Tome III SA: Paris, 1899.

Koch R. Bericht Uber die Thätigkeit der deutschen Cholerakommission in Aegypten und Ostindien. Wien Med Wschr 1883; 33: 1548–1551.

Lakah and Kouri. Sur la fréquence relative des différentes infections conjonctivales aiguës à Alexandrie (Egypte). Ann Oc T 1902; 77: 420–429.

MacCallan AF. Trachoma. Butterworth: London, 1936.

Martin P. Histoire de l'expédition Française en Egypte. Eberhart: Paris, 1855.

Meyerhof M. Über die ansteckenden Augenleiden Ägyptens. Ihre Geschichte, Verbreitung und Bekämpfung. Diemer Nachf. Finck & Baylander: Kairo, 1909.

Onfray R. Comments to a history of French Ophthalmology. Ophthalmologica 134, suppl 32, 1957.

Perthés (editor). Précis des évenéments militaires ou essai historique sur la guerre présente. Tome second. Perthés: Hambourg. Treuttel et Wurtz: Paris et Strasbourg, 1801.

Richardot, lieutenant-colonel. Nouveaux mémoires sur l'armée française en Egypte et en Syrie, ou la vérité mise au jour. Corréard, librairie militaire: Paris, 1848.

Rowe, Huebner et al. Isolation of a cytopathogenic agent from human adenoids undergoing spontaneous degeneration in tissue culture. Proc Soc Exp Biol Med 1953; 84: 570–573.

Weeks J. The bacillus of acute conjunctival catarrh, or 'pink eye'. Arch Opht 1886; 15: 441–451.

Documenta Ophthalmologica 68: 145–156 (1988)

The appointment of Johan Widmark to the first chair in ophthalmology in Stockholm 1891

BJÖRN TENGROTH

Department of Ophthalmology, Karolinska Institute and Hospital, Stockholm, Sweden

The story to be told dates back almost one hundred years. No one still alive can remember this very odd and spectacular academic event far up north in Europe. If the circumstances had been different nothing would have been mentioned, and a rather conventional academic fight would have passed unnoticed.

In the academic world, science in every respect marks daily life. The truth should always be the basis for science, or, at least, what we think is true to the best of our knowledge and mind. But as in religion, where the same fundamental background of truth is thought to be the basis, this truth is different in different parts of the world, in different churches and also different between individuals. It is not accidental that the two scholastic inventions of science and religion have fought each other for centuries. However, as in religion, different opinions of science have fought each other with the same bitterness.

The highest position in the academic world is the professorship, which in the old days always was combined with the chairmanship of a department. This is still true for the non-Anglo-Saxon part of Europe and most of Asia. A professor was, and sometimes still is, looked upon as a person who was far above people in general and the students and younger teachers in particular. The professor could never fail.

This is the necessary background one needs to have to understand the academic fights that have existed for centuries and still exist. When a professor-chair is vacant, the interested doctors will send in their applications to the faculty, and according to European customs not only a board of other professors within the faculty but also a few experts in the actual field will rank the applicants in order to elect the right person. With a sign of great objectivity the ranking list and recommendations are forwarded to the authority that makes the final appointment: The Dean – the Minister – the President – or, in Sweden, the King.

It would be far better if these decisions were made officially subjective as they *de facto* are. As it is now, the air of objectivity often has an odour which

146

is enough to stimulate even rather timid persons to start a bitter fight. The official and "objective" dissection of the applicant's merits resembles an autopsy where the person's bowels and intimate parts are exposed to the public.

In 1888, the Swedish government decided to create an extraordinary chair in ophthalmology at the Karolinska Institute in Stockholm (Fig. 1). The teaching of ophthalmology had up to then been under the responsibility of general surgery, but the importance of the subject, in particular after the invention of the ophthalmoscope by Helmholtz and the fundamental work of von Graefe, Bowman and others, made it evident that an independent chair was a necessity. Two persons, Erik Nordenson and Johan Widmark (Figs. 2–3) sent in their applications. These two persons were entirely different in character, which is of fundamental importance for this story. Some of you might remember the Swedish professor John William Nordenson, who was the honorary president of the world congress in London in 1948.

He was the son of Erik Nordenson, and with his elegance and aristocratic appearance – dressed still in the late 1940s in redingote – he very much resembled his father.

When I try to characterize the combatants I have to base my analysis entirely on what is written and to some small part on what my father – a

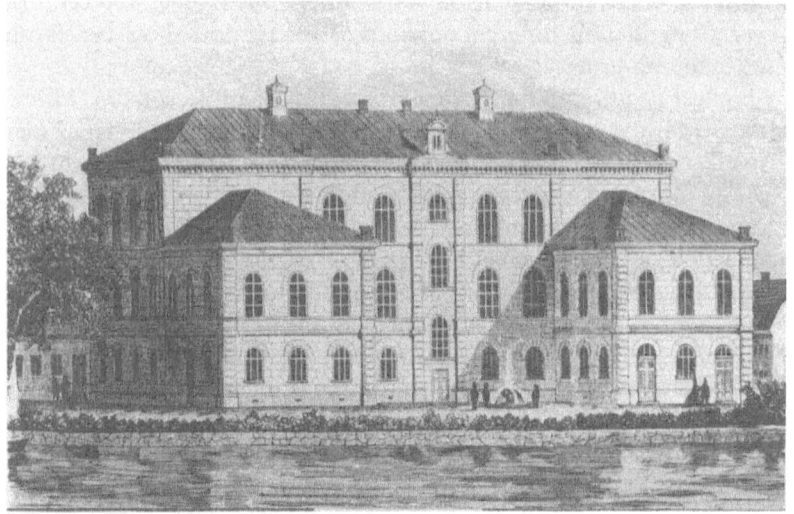

Fig. 1. The Karolinska Institute at the end of the 19th century. From the Karolinska Institute. Ed. B. Pernow, Kugel Printer, Stockholm, 1980.

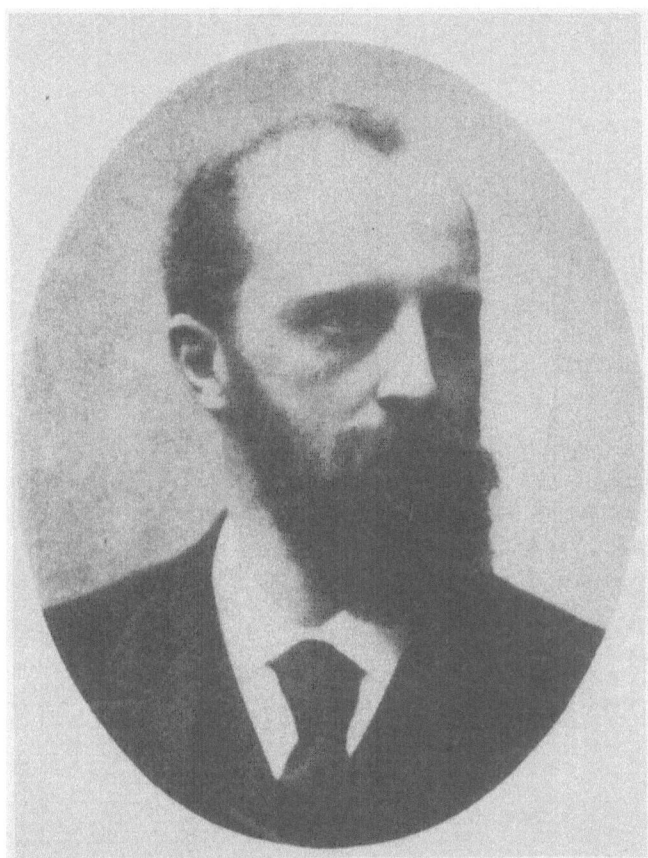

Fig. 2. Dr Erik Nordenson. Private collection photograph.

pupil of J.W. Nordenson's – told me (S. Tengroth, personal communication).

Erik Nordenson was a handsome, elegant man, who could be looked upon as economically independent. He had charisma but could easily be recognized as arrogant and an intellectual snob.

John Widmark was more of a typical academic person with a less marked stature and with a creative mind. He was more of an eager, hard-working person than a society physician.

Although Nordenson spent 9 years after his medical exam working with such giants as Javal, de Wecker, Leber and others, Widmark used 10 months for foreign studies. Most of his time he devoted to work in the laboratory

148

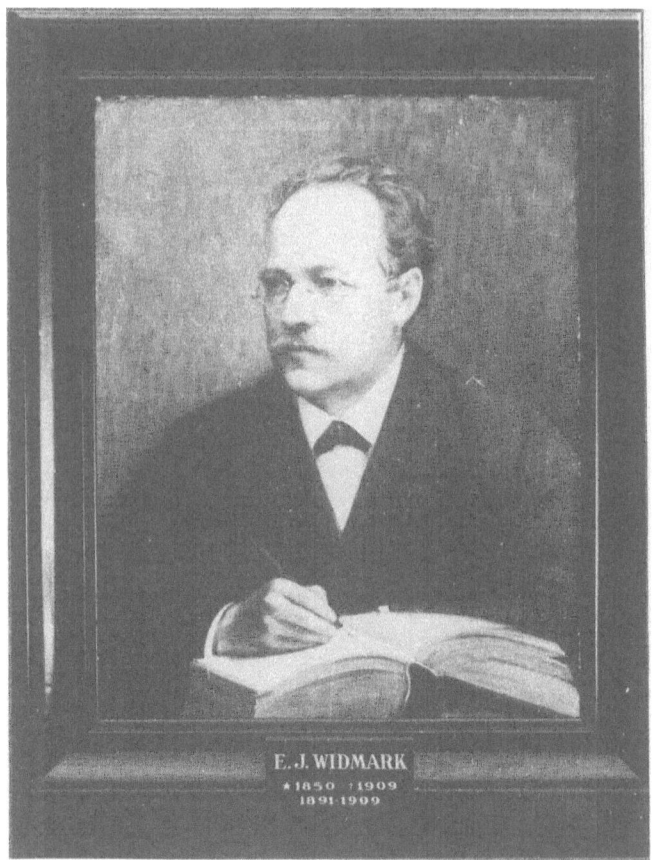

Fig. 3. Prof. E.J. Widmark. Photograph of a painting by Anna Ödmann from the collection of the Eye Clinic, Karolinska Hospital.

and in the clinic. He was also the real teacher in ophthalmology at the Karolinska Institute for a long period.

In 1883 Widmark published and defended his academic thesis on the subject of the "Jequirity-Ophthalmia". In the following years he published a series of scientific papers covering infectious diseases and bacteriology as well as optics. He then started his work on the causes of snow blindness.

With a great knowledge in physics for an ophthalmologist at the time, he was able to prove through a number of rather ingenious experiments that the non-visible short wavelength portion of the spectrum – which he called the ultraviolet part – was responsible for the symptoms and signs of snow blindness. He was also able to characterize the time sequence of the different symptoms, which distinguished them from the symptoms described after exposure to visible violet and blue radiation as well as the signs after exposure to infrared. Reviewing his experimental set-up and his approach to the subject, being somewhat of an expert in the field of non-ionizing radiation myself, I am impressed. There is in my mind no doubt that Widmark was the first scientist to really prove the importance not only of ultraviolet radiation in snow blindness but the importance of this radiation in biology in general. Unlike most of his colleagues at the time he could rule out the so-called chemical radiation which was described as visible violet radiation and point to the fact that ultraviolet radiation is the important and biologically potent exposure factor.

Foucault, Regnault, Charcot and Bouchard among others had described different symptoms in the skin from "chemical radiation", but none had shown that the very specific symptoms in the eye as well as in the skin were caused by the non-visible ultraviolet. Today Widmark is recognized for his fundamental work.

Nordenson, who had studied extensively in all the great clinics of the time, including London, Vienna and Berlin, spent a long time with Javal and de Wecker in Paris and was appointed "directeur adjoint" at the Sorbonne. He then studied for many years with Theodor Leber in Göttingen. During his time in Paris he worked with Javal on the ophthalmometer and investigated a series of school children with this method. His fundamental work, however, was performed in Göttingen. There he investigated 126 cases of retinal detachment from both a clinical and a histological viewpoint and proved one of Leber's theories on the pathogenesis of spontaneous retinal detachment. He stressed the importance of vitreous shrinkage through a series of elegant pathological studies. Even if his work was fully recognized in his time as fundamental, the theory in itself was almost forgotten until recent times, when the importance of the vitreous body in this respect is recognized. Nordenson presented this work for dissertation in 1887 and received the highest mark ever given until then for a thesis at the Karolinska Institute.

In those days the appointment to docent was given to persons with excellent theses almost automatically. Widmark was made docent in 1883, but Nordenson was not given his title until 1889. It was obvious that Nordenson had important enemies in the faculty. That same year the applications were sent to the faculty by Nordenson and Widmark, and the faculty appointed three experts, Professor Rossander from the Institute, Professor Hansen-Grut from Copenhagen, and Dr Hjalmar Schiøtz from Oslo. In 1890, their decision was published. Rossander and Hansen-Grut had written extensively about the eminence of the candidates but placed Widmark before Nordenson, mainly because of his more original scientific work and longer experience as a teacher at the Institute. Schiøtz had only a short notice where he put Nordenson as number one.

The faculty met three times and the discussion was, to say the least, intense. At the May meeting that started in the afternoon, the faculty – at that time 17 members – finished the discussion early in the morning the following day. Five of the members were intimate friends of Nordenson's and signed for him. Unfortunately, Hansen-Grut in his memorandum had some unclear sentences, and as the fight was going on he was accused of misinterpretation of both combatants' works as well as of being biased.

The experts' reports as well as the protocols from the Karolinska Institute's faculty meetings were all published by Nordenson both in Swedish and German [1]. This opened the whole subject to the press and to the public. It was not unusual at the time to publish the details of an academic fight, or at least get parts of the discussion printed and spread among a limited number of people. Nordenson, however, did publish everything including his own analysis of Widmark's papers. In particular he compared Widmark's results and conclusion on the subject of ultraviolet radiation with the scientific work on this particular subject during the previous 50 years. His conclusion was that Widmark had only added a little to what was already known through the work of mainly Foucault, Charcot and Bouchard. Here Nordenson shows that he did not understand this subject and because of that wrongly diminished the importance of Widmark's work.

Perhaps nothing would have happened if Nordenson had not decided to appeal to the King and complain of the unfairness and favouring which in his mind characterized the experts' memoranda as well as the injustice of the majority of the faculty and, as was common in those days, the experts' reports. In his publication Nordenson included a personal conversation with the President of the Institute, Professor Key, which probably was to go too far. In this way he disclosed some of the secrets regarding the handling of similar matters that were common knowledge only of the small group of faculty members and a few persons in the top of the academic world.

An incident of particular interest to illustrate the fierceness of the fight was when the President of the Karolinska Institute, Professor Key, printed a manuscript which dealt not only with the discussion in the faculty but also part of the previously mentioned private discussion between himself and Dr Nordenson. This printed paper was sent from the printer to the Ministry of Justice, as all printed matters in Sweden were at the time. This meant that the government was informed. However, Key did not mean to make this manuscript public, so he went to the Ministry of Justice and through a young and inexperienced clerk he was able to retain his opus. This of course was completely illegal and, as the person who was incriminated was a professor and the president of our most famous medical school, the result was disastrous and poured even more oil on the fire (Figs. 4–5).

As the fight was more and more intense, the newspapers not only in Stockholm but also in the rest of Sweden almost daily had articles on the subject and the "society" as well as the intellectuals of Sweden were divided amongst those for Nordenson and those for Widmark. The fight went on, and Le Figaro, The Times and Neue Züriche Zeitung had a series of articles on the subject.

After a petition from 200 doctors in Sweden (Fig. 6) new experts were appointed: Professor von Hippel of Königsberg, Professor Mauthner of Vienna and Professor Haab of Zürich, so the battlefield was moved to central Europe.

In the summer of 1891, the experts were ready. Von Hippel placed

DOCENT DR. E. NORDENSONS

SCHLUSSBEMERKUNGEN

NEBST EINIGEN BEIGEFÜGTEN ANMERKUNGEN

HERAUSGEGEBEN

VON

JOHAN WIDMARK,
DOCTOR DER MED. UND DOCENT AM KAROL. INSTITUTE.

STOCKHOLM.
1890.

Fig. 4–5. Publications by J. Widmark concerning E. Nordenson's final arguments.

EINIGE WORTE

ANLÄSSLICH

DOCENT DR. ERIK NORDENSONS

SCHLUSSBEMERKUNGEN

VON

JOHAN WIDMARK,

DOKTOR DER MEDICIN UND DOCENT AM KAROLINISCHEN INSTITUT.

———— ◆ — ——

Nordenson as number one and described Widmark's work on snow blindness as a paper on physics. Haab placed Widmark as number one mainly based on his merits as a teacher at the Institute. Mauthner in his memorandum talked highly of Nordenson's work and merits but finished with the following sentence: "Je nach dem Standpunkte, auf welchem die hohen massgebenden Kreise sich befinden, den zu beeinflussen ich jedoch nicht wage, wird die Entscheidung zwischen den beiden Candidaten eine leichte sein". Not until the Foreign Minister of Sweden through the Swedish Ambassador in Vienna had notified Professor Mauthner of a firm decision and sent him the earlier votum of the faculty, did he decide to place Widmark as number one (Fig. 7).

The fight continued with great intensity and almost all important ophthalmologists in Europe were involved. In the Swedish government the ministers were divided but with a slight majority favouring the appointment of Nordenson. The Minister of Education was totally for Nordenson, however, we do not know if it was through friendship or because he was convinced from having studied all the details of the fight.

The King, Oscar II, after long discussions and probably without any possibility of understanding the details of the fight, suddenly made up his

PETITION

SCHWEDISCHER ÄRTZTE

AN

SEINE MAJESTÄT DEN KÖNIG.

Fig. 6. The petition to the King to appoint new experts.

SCHREIBEN

DES KÖNIGL. DEPARTEMENTS DER AUSWÄRTIGEN ANGELEGENHEITEN

AN

DIE GESANDTSCHAFTEN SEINER MAJESTÄT DES KÖNIGS IN BERLIN UND WIEN

UND

DAS GENERALCONSULAT IN GENF,

DAT. STOCKHOLM, DEN 2. JULI 1891.

Fig. 7. The letter from the Foreign Minister to the Swedish Ambassador in Vienna concerning the expert Professor Mauthner.

mind. According to Professor J.W. Nordenson, Dr E. Nordenson's son, the following incident took place.

The Crown Princess Victoria was suffering from an eye disease, and according to her ophthalmologist, who happened to be Nordenson, the disease was a granula uveitis caused by tuberculosis. Even if tuberculosis was a very common disorder at the time among the lower classes, it was recognized as a shameful disease among the upper classes and certainly in the royal family. The King decided to consult a professor and "Geheimrat" in Berlin. The diagnosis according to him was a simple conjunctivitis.

Nordenson was called to the King's chambers and received an admonition for his lack of knowledge, and the King decided against his excellent Minister of Education to appoint Widmark. The minister immediately refused his countersignature and resigned. This resulted in a government crisis.

Nordenson, completely sure of his diagnosis, wrote to his German colleague and asked for an explanation. The following answer arrived: "Entschuldigen Sie, Herr Dozent Nordenson aber ich habe nicht die Kronprinzessin von Schweden in focal Beleuchtung untersucht". He had probably only kissed her hand and given her some eye drops. The Crown Princess and later Queen died many years later from tuberculosis after having spent almost her entire life in Ana Capri because of the climate, and from there her famous personal friend and doctor Munthe published his book on San Michele.

As soon as Widmark was appointed, two of the professors at the Karolinska Institute resigned, and even years later, this fierce animosity was still reflected in different publications. It is said that around 80 publications on this subject were published between the years 1889 and 1892.

A famous inventor and industrialist, a Swede who was brought up in a rich Swedish oil family in Russia, and who among other things invented dynamite – Alfred Nobel – had also a keen interest in medical sciences (Fig. 8).

Together with a Swedish doctor and later professor in physiology at the Karolinska Institute, J.E. Johansson, he started a laboratory for experiments in physiology in Paris. During their collaboration a discussion took place about the vast fortune that Alfred Nobel had collected and what would happen with it, as he had no close family to inherit his money. Johansson had a suggestion that the money should make the basis for a yearly prize in medicine or physiology to a person who had made the most important discovery during the year. The prize winner should be elected by the faculty at the Karolinska Institute. Apparently Nobel accepted this idea and wrote his will. According to J.W. Nordenson (personal communication)

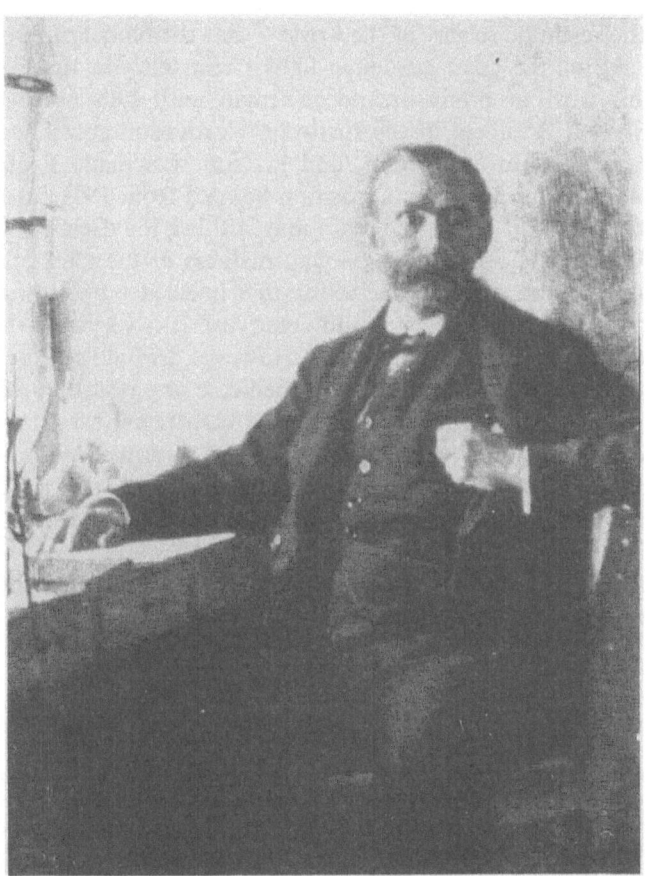

Fig. 8. Alfred Nobel.

Nobel mentioned in 1892 that he could not possibly think of giving the whole fortune to be handled by a faculty which was unable to deal with such a simple matter as to select a professor in ophthamology, so he divided the money to be given as prizes in five different parts. The prize for literature given by the Swedish Academy, two prizes in chemistry and physics through the Royal Academy of Sciences in Stockholm, one prize in medicine or physiology to be given by the faculty of the Karolinska Institute, one prize for peace to be given by the Norska Stortinget – the Norwegian parliament – as Sweden and Norway at the time were united. Today the prize given to the laureates from the hands of his Majesty the King equals US $ 300,000, but it is not the money but the prestige that counts. A prize in medicine of US $ 1,500,000, however of great value, probably would never have had the impact on the scientific society of the world as has the Nobel prize of today.

In the wake of the great academic fight I can tell you that Widmark continued his work as professor and chairman until 1909 and was for a period of 6 years President of the Institute. Nordenson continued with a private eye hospital in Stockholm, and his son was made Professor of Ophthalmology at the Institute, a position he held from 1931 till 1948.

If we had to appoint one of the two today, I think the decision would be the same. Without knowing the personal qualities of the two, other than through the literature, I would like to say that in science two things are of the utmost importance: Excellence and creativity. It is very rare that these two qualities will characterize one person. However, I would say that among the persons selected for the Nobel prize in medicine or physiology during my time in the Nobel Assembly of the Karolinska Institute, most prize winners will fall into this category. When comparing Nordenson and Widmark both could be characterized as excellent, but Widmark also showed a significant amount of creativity which makes the result of his studies still valid. Nordenson's excellent work was based upon Leber's theories and would probably have forwarded vitreous and retinal surgery at a much earlier date, if his work had reflected more of a creative mind.

Reference

1. Nordenson E. Aktenstücke betreffs der Besetzung der ausserordentlichen Professur der Ophthalmologie am Karolinischen Institute. In: Öffentliche Aktenstücke in der Frage von der Besetzung der ausserordentlichen Professur der Ophthalmologie am Karolinischen Institute zu Stockholm. Stockholm, 1892.

Address for offprints: Prof. Björn Tengroth, Dept. of Ophthalmology, Karolinska Hospital, S-104 01 Stockholm, Sweden

Documenta Ophthalmologica 68: 157–169 (1988)

A historical outline of Greek ophthalmology from the Hellenistic period up to the establishment of the first universities

JOHN LASCARATOS & SPIROS MARKETOS

Department of History of Medicine, National University of Athens, Athens, Greece

Abstract. The writers examine the course of Greek ophthalmology from the Hellenistic period to the foundation of the first universities (19th century). In particular, the study refers to Galen, Antyllus, the Byzantine doctors Oribasius, Aetius of Ameda, Paul of Aegina, Alexander of Tralles, Nonnus Theophanes, Theophilus Protospatharius, Michael Psellos, Meletius Monachus, Nemesius bishop of Emeses and John Actuarius. The practice of empirical ophthalmology during the Ottoman domination of Greece is also examined, as is the earliest available evidence of modern Greek ophthalmological knowledge, deriving from the Ionian Islands.

The earliest scientific foundations of ophthalmology are to be discerned in the time of Hippocrates. It is then that medical thinking began to separate itself from the therapeutic views of the Asclepeions and the physical and rational approach to the patient, in accordance with the views of the father of Medicine which also affected the treatment of ophthalmological diseases.

However, the distinction of Ophthalmology as a speciality, (notwithstanding Herodotus' famous passage which indicates the existence of doctors specializing in Ophthalmology in Ancient Egypt (Herodotus, Lib. III, Ch. 84–85, 12–16)) begins later in the Hellenistic period, for it is then that the first foundations in human anatomy and physiology were laid [22]. It is for this reason that our study begins with this period. The classic works of Hirschberg [15] and of Kostomires [21] give a good account of the basic ophthalmological knowledge of the Greeks in pre-Hippocratic times.

Of Hippocrates' successors we should remember Chrysippus (3rd century B.C.) whom several historians consider to be the first surgeon to operate on cataracts [9, 10, 19]. In the same period Evenor of Evepius also thrived and was rewarded with the rights of a hereditary citizen of Athens and a "golden wreath" for "being useful, through his skill, to many of her citizens" [20].

The Alexandrine period is basically represented by Herasistratus and the anatomist Herophilus, who wrote a book dealing specifically with the eyes and to whom we owe many present-day anatomic ophthalmological terms, such as "ragoeides" (uvea), "amphiblestroeides" (retina), "keratoeides" (cornea) and others.

Heliodorus applied himself to the surgery of the eye; Demosthenes Philalethes of Marseilles (40 A.D.) dealt with the opthalmological subjects (fragments of his writings have been preserved in the works of Oribasius and Aetius) and, finally, Gaius also dealt with the eyes [20]. In optics we should remember the work of Euclid.

Most of the writings of ophthalmologists of this period have been lost, but many of their ideas have passed into the works of Galen and of later writers [26].

The work of Galen contains considerable knowledge of the anatomy and physiology of the eye (Galeni, Περί αἰτίας ανμπτ. vol. VII–vol III, Περί χρείας τῶνέν ἀνθρώπον σώματι μορίων, Chap. K).

Galen [13] describes four coats of the eye, the cornea (with the sclera), the uvea (or ragoeides), the retina and the conjunctiva and three "humours", the vitreous humour, the crystalline humour (lens) and the aqueous humour and recognizes 7 of the 12 cerebral nerves. Remarkable also is his knowledge of the correct position of the lens, which was "rediscovered" during the Renaissance by Fabricius ab Aquapendente (1533–1619) [23]. He is acquainted with a great number of eye diseases (Galeni, vol. XIV, "Εἰσαγωςῆ ἥ" Ιατρός" and Vol. XIX, ᾽ατρικοί ὅροι) and has considerable knowledge of ophthalmological medicaments. He recommends a wide selection of collyria (eye-drops) for different maladies of the eyes [13], which he names after their original makers such as, for instance, "the collyrion of Gaius the ophthalmologist", "the collyrion of Zoilus", Colyrion of Asclepiades Pakkius for eye pain, of Phoenix Apollonius et al. as well as several collyria of his own invention (Galeni, vol XII, Περί ουνθέσεως φαρμάκων τῶν κατά τόπους, books D and E and vol. XIV, "Περί εὐπορίστων", books A, B and C, "Πρός τά τοῦ ὀφθαλμοῦ," Ch. E).

He even recommends surgical treatment of eye diseases [13] (Galeni, XIV, ἰσαγωγή ἥ ᾽Ιατρός) such as trichiasis, pterygium, hypochyma, staphyloma, eganthis, aegylops and proposes paracentesis for hypopyon. In addition, Galen makes broad references to the theories concerning vision that had been elaborated up to his days, and, significantly, analyses the fundamental importance of the lens and lays the foundations of binocular vision with the theory of geometric lines and cones [13] (Galeni, XIX, "Περί Φιλοσόφου ᾽Ιστορίας" ch. ςέ. "Περί ὀράσεως καί πῶς ὀρῶμες", Vol. III, "Περί χρείας τῶν ἐν ἀνθρώπου σώμπου σώματι μορίων, ch. k').

Though Galen's writings dealing specifically with ophthalmology have not been preserved, we know of the following: "Optici logi" (Οπτικοί λόγοι), "The diagnosis of eye diseases", "Treatise on the treatment of all

Table 1. Ophthalmic diseases mentioned by Aetius.

I Eyelids	IV Disturbances of vision
emphysema	myopia
oedema	amblyopia
phlyctena	presbyopia
symblepharon	amaurosis
phthiriasis	nyctalopia
trichiasis – distichiasis	
sclerophthalmia	V Anterior chamber – pupil – lens
xerophthalmia	hypopyon
psorophthalmia	glaucosis
madarosis	hypochyma
apostema	mydriasis
lithiasis	phthisis of the pupil (= miosis)
chalazion	
hordeolum	VI Inflammation of the lacrimal
steatoma	ducts
varicosis	aegilops
anthrax	anchylops
II Cornea	VII Traumas – burns
ulcer (Bothrion-coeloma)	trauma
phlyctena	foreign bodies
argemon – nebula – achlys –	chemical burns
epicauma – eccauma	thermal burns
leucoma	
staphyloma	VII Miscellaneous
cancerous ulcer	proptosis
	phthisis bulbi
III Sclera – Conjunctiva	lagophthalmos
ophthalmia – taraxis	paralysis of the eye
phlyctena	
subconjunctival hemorrhages	
ulcer	
trachoma – sycosis – tyle	
hemorrhages of the canthus	
pinguecula	
eganthis	
rhyas ($\rho\nu\acute{\alpha}\varsigma$ = epiphora)	

ophthalmic diseases", and, finally, the book on surgery in which he describes, as he himself mentions elsewhere, the surgical method for the extraction of the hypochyma [2, 3, 15].

A contemporary of Galen, Antyllus, was a great surgeon. He is best known for his description of the surgical treatment of aneurysms which remained a classic till the time of John Hunter. At the same time, however, he applied himself to eye surgery, and particularly to plastic surgery on colobomas of the eyelid and the extraction (!) and suction of cataracts, as

160

Table 2. Surgical diseaess of the eye mentioned by Aetius.

---

staphyloma
pinguecula (?)
pterygium
eganthis
blepharon
trichiasis
ectropion (operations method of Demosthenes and Antyllos)
lagophthalmos
chalazion
hordeolum
steatoma
aegilops
anchylops

---

we know from the famous passage by Rhazes, which has caused great controversy among historians, as it indicates that Antyllus was the first proponent of the extraction of cataracts, centuries before the method was established by Daviel [14, 16, 17, 28].

Furthermore, Antyllus recommends several collyria for eye ailments. Fragments of his works are known to us from Spregel (1799) and from Oribasius (Ed. Bussemaker – Daremberg, Paris 1851–1876). Even before Galen and Antyllus, Rufus Ephesius (98–117 A.D.), in his treatise "Concerning the position and nomenclature of human parts" (Ed. Clinch 1726 and Daremberg 1879) and in fragments of his other works which have been preserved through Oribasius and Rhazes, had, relying on the discoveries of the Alexandrine period, not only given an anatomic description of the eye and recognized 44 different eye ailments, but had been the first to distinguish between glaucosis and hypochyma [36, 37].

Of the later Byzantine doctors, we shall deal mainly with Oribasius, Aetius of Ameda, Paul of Aegina and Alexander of Tralles. Aetius (6th century A.D.), personal physician to Justinian I, was, of course, a compiler, but what stands out is the discernment shown in his choice of medical texts. In the opinion of Neuburger and Hirschberg his description and classification of ophthalmic diseases is the most comprehensive and remarkable of his age.

The seventh chapter of his work, entitled "Concerning Maladies of the Eye" [1], comprises the anatomy of the eye, a description of 61 eye diseases together with the pharmacological and surgical treatment of each (Tables 1 and 2) – (Ed. Olivieri).

Many of his topics originate in the works of Demosthenes, of Galen, Philagrius, Dioscorides, Antyllus and Seberus. Of particular interest is the

Table 3. Diseases of the eye mentioned by Oribasius.

ophthalmia
chemosis
phlyctena
anthrax (of the eyelids)
phthiriasis
phthisis bulbi
nyctalopia
mydriasis
glaucoma – hypochyma
amaurosis – amblyopia
strabismus
myopia
epiphora
eganthis
synchysis (of the vision)

Table 4. Ophthalmic diseases mentioned by Paul of Aegina.

taraxis – ophthalmia (conjunctivitis)
chemosis
subconjunctival hemorrhages
emphysema –oedema (of the eyelids)
psorophthalmia
sclerophthalmia and xerophthalmia
ectropion
aegilops and anchylops
trachoma
chalazion
hordeolum
phthiriasis
madarosis
ptilosis
eganthis – rhyas
ulcer
proptosis
hypopyon
leucoma
pterygium
anthrax
carcinoma of the cornea (= ulcer)
mydriasis
phthisis
nyctalopia
glaucoma – hypochyma
strabismus
synchysis
myopia

Table 5. Surgical diseases of the eye mentioned by Paul of Aegina.

lagophthalmos
ectropion
entropion – trichiasis
symblepharon
chalazion
eganthis
staphyloma
hypochyma
aegilops
cysts
verrucae

fact that nowhere does he mention the surgical treatment of cataracts by Aetius but refers only to pharmaceutical treatment.

Alexander of Tralles (525–605? A.D.) though considered a disciple of the Galenic tradition, added several findings of his own, mainly to descriptions of eye diseases and treatments. What interested him most was pathology and therapeutics but at the same time "he dealt with the greatest attention with diseases of the eye" (p5).

Oribasius (325–403 A.D.), friend and physician to Julian the Apostate, faithfully follows Galen, though on many points he relies on Demosthenes, Rufus, Archigenes, Antyllus, Apuleus of Pergamon, Aristotle, Asclepiades and Soranus [5].

Despite their compilatory character, his works are of value for he selects those opinions of ancient doctors that are most correct for his age, and today the original works he refers to have been lost. His "Collections" were the "Encyclopaedia of Medicine" of his time.

From the ophthalmological point of view, he concerned himself with the anatomy of the eye (Bussemaker-Daremberg, Vol. 3, Ch.d, On the eye, "Des yeux"; Ch. $\kappa\eta$', On muscles of the eye, "Des muscles de l'oeil"; ch. $\kappa\vartheta$', On the muscles which move the eyelid, "Des muscles qui meuvent les Paupières") prescribed a series of collyria (Vol. 5, "Des Médicaments Composés") and described several ailments of the eye [30] (Vol. 5, "Maladies des Yeux", Synopsis VIII) – (Table 30).

The ophthalmological work of the last great Byzantine doctor, Paul of Aegina (625–690 A.D.) may be found in the third and sixth book of his writings (Ed. Aldus). The third book describes maladies of the eye [31] (table 4). The value of Paul of Aegina's work, however, stems from his chapter on surgery which indicates that the technical skill of the surgeons of the age had reached such perfection as to enable them to carry out, with remarkable success, such difficult and delicate operations as hernias (which operation

Table 6. Ophthalmic diseases mentioned by Nonnus Theophanis.

distichiasis
trichiasis
chalazion
taraxis – ophthalmia
chemosis
subconjunctival hemorrhage
emphysema
psoriasis
sclerophthalmia and xerophthalmia
ectropion
aegilops and anchylops
milphosis
rhyas
ulcer (of the cornea) (Bothrion-coeloma-argemon-epicauma)
trichiasis
staphyloma
amaurosis
glaucosis – hypochyma
epiphora
leucoma
pterygium
amblyopia
nyctalopia
anthrax
carcinoma
hypopyon

remained a classic up to the end of the 17th Century), the removal of haemorrhoids, condylomas, and varicose veins, as well as lithothrypty, castration etc.

In his sixth book [31], which is the most important in that it provides a clear picture of the progress made in surgery from the time of Celsus to his own day, he explains the surgical technique of ophthalmological operations for the following 12 diseases (Table 5).

Nonnus Theophanes, in his "Epitome" [29] deals with the treatment of several eye diseases, after first providing a brief definition of each. His treatise therefore, may be considered a therapeutic guide to ophthalmology of his times. First of all, he prescribes medicaments "to thicken the eyebrows" and "to darken the eyebrows" (Ch. MA′ and MB′). Then (Ch. MΓ′-OΓ′) he prescribes for the following 33 diseases (Table 6) – (Ed. Bernard). A whole chapter is devoted to collyria (Ch. ΞA′).

A contemporary of Paul of Aegina, Theophilus Protospatharius, who was an officer and physician to the emperor Heraclius (603–645 A.D.) examines human anatomy and physiology from a teleologic, religious point of view.

164

Table 7. Ophthalmic diseases mentioned by Leon Philosophi.

xerophthalmia
phthisis bulbi
trachoma – sycosis
chalazion
hordeolum
lithiasis (of the eyelids)
phthiriasis
trichiasis
phalogosis (= Distichiasis –tristichiasis)
ptilosis (or ptosis)
paralysis (of the eyelids)
eganthis
rhyas
pterygium
symblepharon (or prosphysis or symphysis)
aegilops
subconjunctival hemorrhage (Hyposphagma or aematis)
chemosis
argemon
nephelion – achlys – leucoma
hypopyon
ulcers of the cornea (Bothrion-Myocephalon)
staphyloma
hypochyma
myxriasis (or ptatycoria)
glaucosis
synchysis
symptosis (miosis)
paremptosis
nyctalopia
ectropion
cysts
hypopyon

His work "Concerning the structure of the human body" (De Corporis Humani Fabrica) – (Ed. Guilielmus Alexander Greenhill) devotes a separate chapter to the anatomy of the eye (and the first cerebral nerve) and to the function of vision [38].

Leon, the philosopher and doctor, in his work "Conspectus Medicinae" elaborates on the anatomy of the eye and of the optical nerve, which, in accordance with the Galenic view, he considers to be the only hollow nerve, so that "the spirit of vision" may pass through it to the eyes. He also makes particular mention of the chiasma opticum (beginning of chapter three) [24]. At the same time, he deals with the definition and treatment of 37 diseases (Table 7) – (Ed. Ermerins).

Michael (Constantine) Psellos (1020–1105 A.D.), "The Greatest of Philosophers" as he was called by the emperor Constantine Monomachis [12], gives in his "Medical Treatise", an iambic poem of 1372 lines, a definition in verse form, of taraxis, ophthalmia, chemosis, hyposphagma, emphysema, psorophthalmia, xerophthalmia, ectropion, trachoma-sycosis, chalazion, hordeolum, milphosis, eganthis, rhyas, proptosis (staphyloma, helon, myocephalon etc.), leucoma, pterygium, Carcinoma of the cornea, anthrax, mydriasis, miosis (phthisis), nyctalopia, glaucosis, hypochyma, amblyopia, amaurosis and strabismus (Ed. Olms) [35].

Meletius Monachus (4th Century A.D.), a monk at the monastery of the Holy Trinity at Tiberopoli, includes a special chapter "Concerning the Eyes" (Ch.b) in his "De Natura Hominis" in which, after first expressing his wonder at the divine work he supplies information on the anatomy of the eye, the function of vision and colour perception [25] (Ed. Migne).

Meletius' book is a summary of previous medical knowledge and contains nothing new. The writer's purpose was to collect together scattered pieces of knowledge from the works of Galen, Socrates, The Great Baselius, Gregory Chrysostome, Cyril and others [11, 12, 25].

Nemesius, Bishop of Emeses, in Syria (4th–5th Century A.D.), in his work "On Human Nature" (De Natura Hominis, Ed. Migne), which is remarkable for its physiology of the nervous system, refers more thoroughly to the matter of visual function [27].

Byzantine medicine came to a glorious end, according to Neuburger, with the work of John Actuarius, son of Zacharias, concerning the diagnosis and treatment of various diseases, uroscopy and psychopathology.

In his dealings with ophthalmological subjects we may discern, not a simple enumeration of material, but the working of a spirit of differential diagnosis [18].

In his chapter "On Ophthalmological Diagnosis" (John Actuaris, De Diagnosi, Lib. II, Ch. j') he deals with the following illnesses which he explains from the point of view of differential diagnosis (Table 8). (The illnesses for which he provides differential diagnosis are listed in Table 8 in the same order).

Finally, we should mention Pedacius Dioscorides (54–68 A.D.) who mentions, in his "De medica Materia" [8] (Ed. I. Soteris), the therapeutic treatment for several maladies of the eye.

From what we have so briefly mentioned, it appears that Byzantine medicine, while not adding spectacular discoveries or original elements, safeguarded the heritage of the ancient Greek doctors for posterity.

The contribution of Arabic medicine to the medical thinking of the West was of a comparable nature.

166

Table 8. Diseases of the eye mentioned by Ioannes Actuarius.

taraxis – ophthalmia – epiphora of the rheuma
subconjunctival hemorrhage
chemosis
psorophthalmia – xerophthalmia
ectropion
aegilops
trachoma – sycosis – tyle – chalazion – hordeolum
phthiriasis
madarosis (milphosis)
trichosis (= trichiasis)
eganthis – rhyas
ulcer (of the cornea) – epicauma
argema
proptosis (staphyloma etc.)
hypopyon
nebula – leucoma
pterygium
anthrax – carcinoma
mydriasis – phthisis (miosis) – phthisis bulbi
nyctalopia
glaucoma – hypochyma
strabismus
myopia

After the fall of Byzantium, scientific medicine, and consequently ophthalmology declined in the Greek speaking world. Throughout the centuries of Ottoman domination ophthalmology was doomed to take on the empirical characteristics of medical practice in general, the characteristics of charlatanism, of the "Kombogiannites".

A remnant of this kind of "practical" ophthalmology is the couching of the lens which used to be carried out by lay ophthalmologists at Kravara (modern-day Naupactos) until shortly after the Second World War.

The very same example, however, proves something more: that ancient Greek medical tradition, in an altered form perhaps, passed into the hands of these empirical doctors. For the method of couching is the very same ancient method, taught to us in detail by Paul of Aegina, Galen and other ancient writers. After the fall of Constantinople, the Byzantine doctors who fled to Europe must have practiced ophthalmology. Evidence of this, which, however, requires further study, is provided in the writings of the son of a Byzantine refugee in Messene, Francis Maurolykus (1497–1577) who was the first to realize that the retina is the main organ of vision [4]. As for the free parts of the Greek speaking world, the information we have concerning the 15th century is negligible, while it is limited concerning the 16th.

The first doctors, in the Ionian Islands, who had studied in Padua, returned to their homelands in the mid 17th century. Up to that time, we have to suppose, medical practice had been of an empirical nature, for no contrary written evidence exists [32, 33].

From the very first years of the occupation of the islands by the Venetians there existed a number of doctors who practiced empirical medicine, and in 1566 a "Hospitale" (Spitalio) was established in the Castle of Cephalonia.

The first evidence available concerning the practice of ophthalmology in the Ionian Islands dates from 1637. Misser (Monsieur) Cristodoulos Padovanos (whose name shows him to be a foreigner) was not only the first ophthalmologist (empirical apparently) in Cephalonia, but had such confidence in his healing powers that he signed a contract in which he promised "to cure the above-mentioned Master Niko (Paramythiotes) of the weak vision in his eyes within a term of three months and, on being cured, the above-mentioned master Niko to be under obligation to pay the same Misser Cristodoulos a sum of twenty (20) reals for the cure, and in the case that he is not cured, not to be under obligation to pay him anything" [32].

A second piece of written evidence of Ionian ophthalmology is much more recent and dates from the 18th century (7th Dec. 1757). It was published by Leonid Zoes in the magazine "The Muses" of Zante, and again by Charamis in the Bulletin of the Hellenic Ophthalmological Society [6]. It consists of an affirmation by the foreign ophthalmologist Anastasius Kotzie certifying that Antony Rouzmeles of Zante studied "medicine of the eyes" under him. This is the first known speciality diploma, though, of course, on a private basis.

Even in the times of the Ionian Academy (1824–1828, 1844–1865) ophthalmology does not appear as a separate lecture in the syllabuses of the time which have been preserved, though it was probably a part of lectures on surgery, as was the general practice of the day.

There is, however, an important piece of evidence which permits us to suppose that the Ionian Academy showed interest in ophthalmology.

This document, which was located by Ass. Professor G. Pentogalos in the Archives of the Ionian State, is a report by Nikolaos Maratos, a professor at the Ionan Academy, submitted to Lord Guildford who passed it on, on 5th April 1826, to the Secretariat of the Senate [34].

Professor Maratos, proposed the purchase, among other things, of the surgical ophthalmological instruments belonging to the great teacher of the nation, Athanasius Psallidas (1760–1833) [7].

Apart from the exception of the Ionian Academy, however, the practice of ophthalmology in the rest of Greece must have remained all those years within the framework of empirical medicine, at least until the establishment of the first Greek University.

References

1. Aetii Amideni. Libri medicinales V–VIII, Ed. Alexander Olivieri. Berolini in Aedibus Academiae Litterarum, 1950.
2. Anagnostakis A. Contributions à l'histoire de la chirurgie oculaire chez les anciens. Athènes: Perris Frères, 1872.
3. Anagnostakis A. Encore deux mots sur l'extraction de la cataracte chez les anciens. Anthènes: P. Perris, 1878.
4. Arrington EG. A History of Ophthalmology. New York: M.D. Publications, 1959; 74.
5. Castiglioni A. History of Medicine. Athens, 1961.
6. Charamis IS. A historical note concerning an Ophthalmologist of Zante in the 18th century. Bull of the Hellenic Ophthalmological Society 1950; 18: 30–31.
7. Chiotis P. Historical memoirs of the Ionian Islands. Vol 7. Athens: Karavias, 1981.
8. Dioscoridae Pedacii Anazarbei, De Medica Materia Libri V etc., Coloniae, Opera et imprensa Ioannis Soteris, 1709.
9. Esser MA. Zu Knapps Mitteilung von der Staroperation bei den alten Griechen. Klin Mbl Augenheilk 1931; 86: 679.
10. Esser A. Weiteres zur ältesten Kenntnis der Katarakt-Operation. Klin Mbl Augenheilk, 1956; 129: 396–404.
11. Gabrielides A. About medical knowledge and especially about the eye according to the Byzantine writers, Hellenic Literary Associations of Constantinople. Biological Committee. Meeting of 29 November 1908; 28: 92–102.
12. Gabrielides A. About the Ophthalmological knowledge of the Byzantine writers and about the term "Nyctalops". Hellenic Literary Association of Constantinople. Biological Committee. Meeting of 10 February 1908; 28: 53–62.
13. Galeni Claudii. Opera Onnia. D. Carolus Gottlob Kühn. Lipsiae. Vol III (1822), pp 759–814, Vol VII (1824), pp 725–823, Vol. XII (1826), Vol XIV (1827), pp 339–501, 783–784, Vol XIX (1830) pp 306–309, 358–439.
14. Garrison FH. An introduction to the history of medicine. Philadelphia and London: Saunders, 1929.
15. Hirschberg J. Geschichte der Augenheilkunde. In: Graefe A, Saemisch ET, eds. Handbuch der gesamten Augenheilkunde, zwölfter Band. Leipzig: Wilhelm Engelmann, 1899.
16. Hirschberg J. Die Star-Operation nach Antyllos. Centralblatt für Praktische Augenheilkunde 1906; April: 98–100.
17. Hirschberg J. Zur Geschichte der Star-Operation. Centralblatt für Praktische Augenheilkunde. 1906a. Mai: 133–135.
18. Ideler LI. Physici et Medici Graeci minores, Vol II. Berolini, G. Reimeri, 1842: 444–449.
19. Knapp P. Zur Frage der Staroperation bei den alten Griechen. Klin Mbl Augenheilk 1930; 84: 277–299.
20. Kouzis A. History of medicine. Athens, 1929.
21. Kostomires G. About ophthalmology and otology among the ancient Greeks from ancient times until Hippocrates. Athens, 1887.
22. Lascaratos J, Marketos S. From the History of glaucoma and cataract. Greek Annals of Ophthalmology 1981; 18: 219–241.
23. Lascaratos J, Marketos S. The cataract operation in Ancient Greece. Histoire des Sciences Médicales 1982; 17: 317–322.
24. Leonis Philosophi et Medici. Conspectus Medicinae. Anecdota Medica Graeca. Amsterdam: FZ. Ermerins, AM Hakkert, 1963: 127–151.
25. Meletii Monach. De Natura Hominis, Ch. b, About the Eyes. Paris: I.-P. Migne, 1860; 64: 1161–1169.

26. Meyer-Steineg Th, Sudhoff K. Geschichte der Medizin im Überblick mit Abbildungen. Jena: Gustar Fischer, 1922; 34–92 (Zweite Auflage).
27. Nemesii Episcopi Emeseni. De Natura Hominis, About the Vision. Paris: I.-P. Migne, 1858; 40: 637–649.
28. Neuburger M. History of medicine, Vol I. London: Oxford University Press, 1910.
29. Nonni Theophanis. Epitome de Curatione Morborum Graece ac Latine etc. Vol I, Gothae – Amstelodami, I.O. Steph. Bernard 1794, pp 186–189, 190–263,234–236.
30. Oribase. Oeuvres d'Oribase etc. Vol V. Paris: Bussemaker et Ch. Daremberg, 1873; Vol III, pp. 294–304, 424–428. Vol V. pp. 132–141, 441–459.
31. Pauli Aeginetae Medici Optimi. Libri Septem etc. Venetiis, Aldus, 1528.
32. Pentogalos G. The oldest known information concerning medical and infirmary treatment in Cefalonia. Athens, 1974.
33. Pentogalos G. The views of the Arab Doctor Imn Al Tzazzar (920–1009) concerning internal medicine and therapeutics. From his book "Ephodia" included in the manuscript of the Corgialenios Library of Argostoli. Argostoli, 1974a.
34. Pentogalos G. The Medical School of Ionian Academy (1824–1828 and 1844–1865). Thessaloniki, 1980.
35. Psellos. Medical Treatise, Anecdota Graeca etc. Vol I. Fr. Boissonade, Hildesheim, Georg Olms Verlagsbuchhandlung, 1962; 210–212.
36. Rufus of Ephesus. Περί τῶν ἐν κύστει καί νεφροῖς παϑροῖς παϑῶς etc. Londini: Gulielmus Clinch, 1726.
37. Rufus d'Ephèse. Oeuvres de Rufus D'Ephèse texte collationné sur les manuscrits traduit pour la première fois en Français. Paris: Ch. Daremberg, 1879.
38. Theophili Protospatharil. De Corporis Humani Fabrica, Libri V. Oxonii, Guilielmus Alexander Greenhill, 1842: 150–174.

Archive sources

1. Historical Archives of Corfu. Archives of the Ionian State. Document of Lord Guilford to secretary of the Senate S. Osborne. 20/193 (5-4-1826).
2. Historical Archives of Cefalonia. Notary's Archives. Documents of Notary Raphael Piniatorre (1635–1649). Book 1635–1642, Document dated 4 July 1637.

Documenta Ophthalmologica 68: 171–176 (1988)
© Kluwer Academic Publishers, Dordrecht

History of the Japanese Ophthalmological Society

AKIRA NAKAJIMA[1] & SHIZU SAKAI[2]
[1]*Dept. of Ophthalmology, Juntendo School of Medicine, Japan;*
[2]*Dept. of Medical History, Juntendo School of Medicine, Japan*

Introduction

In Chinese traditional medicine, ophthalmology is a part of the speciality on five sense organs, and is not an independent one. Ophthalmology and otorhinolaryngology used to be one speciality in countries with British tradition. In the USA, ophthalmology and otorhinolaryngology have formed separate societies only since a few years. In many other countries, ophthalmology used to be a separate and independent speciality of clinical medicine.

The Japanese Ophthalmological Society celebrated its 90th anniversary in 1986. It was founded on 27 February, 1897 in Tokyo. As a medical society in Japan, it is among the oldest besides the Society of Forensic Medicine (founded in 1887), the Society of Medical History (founded in 1892), the Anatomical Society and the Society of Otorhinolaryngology (founded in 1893). It is the second oldest society in clinical medicine in Japan, followed by the Society of Surgery founded in 1898, the Society of Obstretrics and Gynecology (1901), the Society of Gastroenterology (1902), the Society of Internal Medicine (1903), etc. It seems that the foundation of the Ophthalmological and the Otorhinolaryngological Societies has triggered the foundation of many other societies of clinical medicine.

The foundation of the Japanese Ophthalmological Society

In Japan, ophthalmology became a separate and independent speciality of medicine already in the 15th century. The early development of ophthalmology was furthered in Japan early in the 19th century by several European doctors, especially by Dr. Pompe, the pupil of Prof. Donders in the Netherlands. In addition, Japan adopted the German system of medicine just after the Meiji Revolution of 1857. In Germany, ophthalmology has been an independent speciality since the era of von Graefe, and the German Ophthalmological Society, founded in 1863, is the oldest ophthalmological society in the world besides the International Ophthalmological Congress which first convened in 1857. It is no wonder then, that the Japanese Ophthalmological Society was founded under a strong German influence. Preceding activities in Japanese ophthalmological circles lead to the foundation of the Japanese Ophthalmological Society. Several eye hospitals were opened soon after the Meiji Revolution, much earlier than the hospitals of other specialities. It is ironical that, even now, we have only private eye hospitals and no independent public eye hospital or institute in Japan, even though private eye hospitals have been created very early in the history of modern medicine in Japan. A study group in ophthalmology was organized in 1884 under the leadership of Kinnojo Ume, the first professor of Ophthalmology in Japan at the University of Tokyo. It did not last more than one year because of the premature death of Prof. Ume. Another study group in ophthalmology was organized in 1889 by Tatsuya Inoue (1848–1895; Fig. 1)

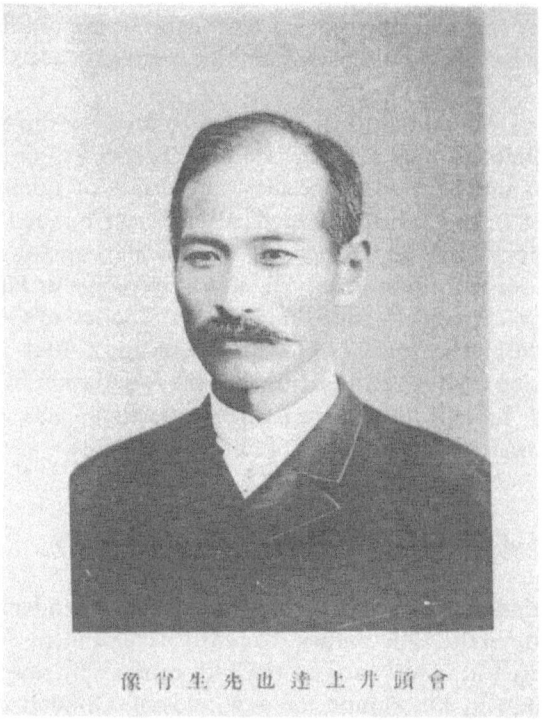

Fig. 1. Portrait of Dr. Tatsuya Inoue (1848–1895).

at the Inoue Eye Hospital in Tokyo. Reports of the Inoue Ophthalmic study group were published until the accidental death of Dr. Tatsuya Inoue, the leader of the group, at the age of 49.

There were several important figures in the foundation of the Japanese Ophthalmological Society, but the most important was undoubtedly Yoshiakira Onishi (1865–1932). He studied ophthalmology in Germany, and came back to Japan in 1890. He started, with fourteen other ophthalmologists, an ophthalmic journal called "Ganka (ophthalmology) Zasshi (journal)" in July, 1893 (Fig. 2). However, the journal did not continue appearing beyond volume 3, number 2. It had to stop publication in 1896 mainly because of the lack of articles for publication.

In the meantime, Takuji Suda (1869–1941) came back from Germany in 1894. Yoshiakira Onishi, Takuji Suda and Motojiro Kawakami (Fig. 3) came together to discuss the future of ophthalmology in Japan. They agreed

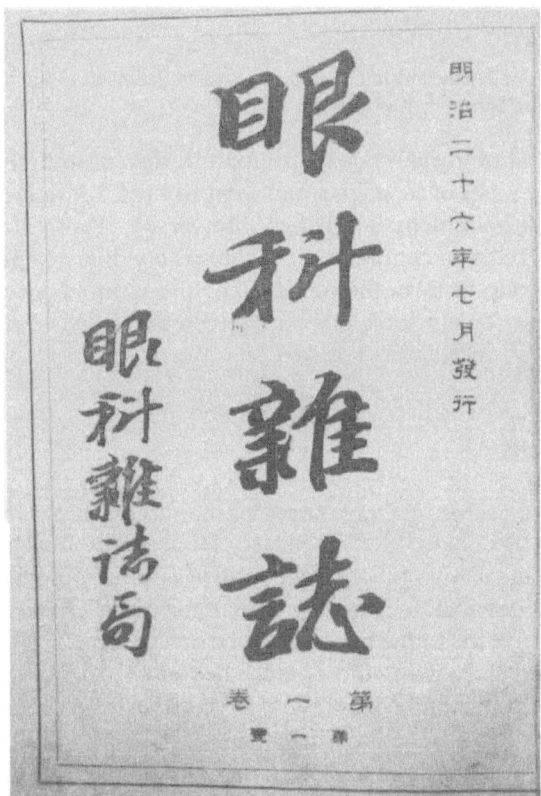

Fig. 2. Cover of Ganka Zasshi vol. 1 No. 1, published in July 1893.

174

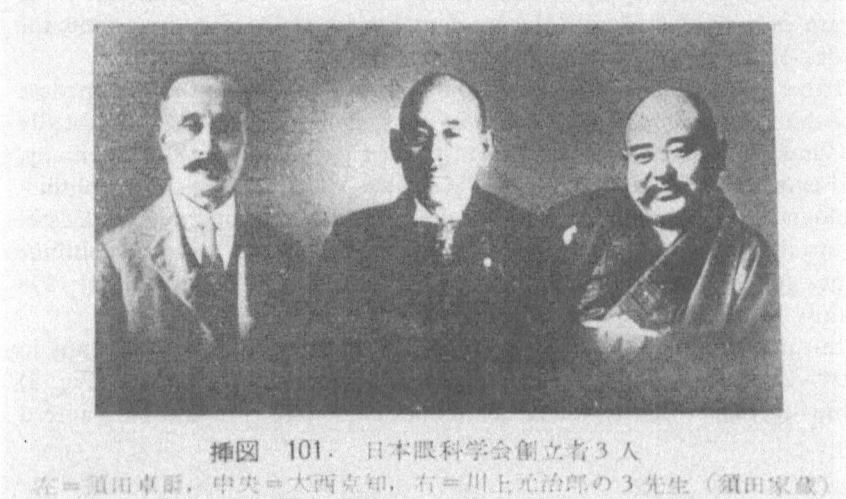

挿図 101. 日本眼科学会創立者3人
左＝須田卓爾，中央＝大西克知，右＝川上元治郎の3先生（須田家蔵）

Fig. 3. Three founders of Japanese Ophthalmological Society (from left to right: Takuji Suda, Yoshiakira Onishi, and Motojiro Kawakami).

to form an ophthalmological society in Japan in the autumn of 1896. They obtained the agreement of colleagues and went to Prof. Jujiro Komoto, then professor of ophthalmology at Tokyo University. Prof. Komoto first doubted the possibility of continuation of the society, but was persuaded by Onishi and his group to form the society. The preparatory meeting for the foundation of the society took place in December, 1896 in a restaurant called "Mikawaya" in Kanda, Tokyo.

The Inaugural Congress

The Inaugural Congress of the Japanese Ophthalmological Society was held for three days at the Tokyo Medical Society House, Nihonbashi, Tokyo on 27, 28 February and 1 March, 1897. Ninety-five ophthalmologists attended. The first day was devoted to ceremony of inauguration. The morning of the second day was devoted to the business of the newly formed society, discussion of bylaws and election of officers, etc. The morning of the third day was spent visiting eye clinics and hospitals for the demonstration of patients and surgeries.

The afternoon of the second and third day was devoted to the reporting of papers. In all, 18 papers were read at the first congress. The program is listed in Table 1. The papers as well as the inaugural business are recorded in the inaugural issue (No. 1–4 inclusive) of Acta Societatis Ophthalmologicae Japonicae, published in April, 1897 (Fig. 4). Since then, the society's annual congress has been held regularly with the exception of two occasions: in 1905 because of the Japan-Russia War, and from 1944 to 1945 because of the Second World War.

The present and future of the Society

The society has grown in activities as well as in size. During the past 90 years, the members have grown from 95 in 1897 to over 7000 in 1986, working for the eye health of Japanese people using 2 billion US dollars per year. It installed an ophthalmologist specialist qualification system in 1982. The ophthalmologists qualified by the Society will be born in Japan in 1989. After 1989 there will be 300 and 400 newly qualified ophthalmologists expected annually.

The Japanese Ophthalmological Society became a member of the International Federation of Ophthalmological Societies in 1935. Japanese ophthalmologists have taken part in the International Congresses of Ophthalmology since 1929 at the 13th Congress held in Amsterdam. It

Table 1. Papers read at the Inaugural Congress of Japanese Ophthalmological Society.

Afternoon on 28 February, 1897.	
On cataract surgery.	Shunkichi Miyashita.
Point of gaze in visual field measurement.	Tsubasa Yamashita.
Visual impairment related to oxalic aciduria.	Ninzaburo Watari.
On so-called subconjunctival injection.	Seijira Iesaka.
Sugery for ptosis.	Jujiro Komoto.
Cataract surgery.	Juriro Komoto.
Surgical treatment of trachoma.	Kokuchi Onishi.
Afternoon on 1st March.	
On cataract surgery.	Kazuaki Kato.
Demonstration of a case of lid convulsion.	Takuji Suda.
Surgery for myopia.	Minosuke Kuniya.
A case of iritis.	Koan Miyazaki.
600 cases of intraocular iron foreign body.	Jiro Akino.
Treatment of traumatic scleral wound.	Buichiro Kurokawa.
A case of hyaline degeneration of conjunctiva.	Tasuku Kono.
Surgery for entropium and trichiasis of the lid.	Kyoji Kiribuchi.
Microscopic findings of conjunctival scrapings of blenorrhoea.	Atsushi Hijikata.
Spontaneous bleeding of orbit.	Tsugishige Kondo.

176

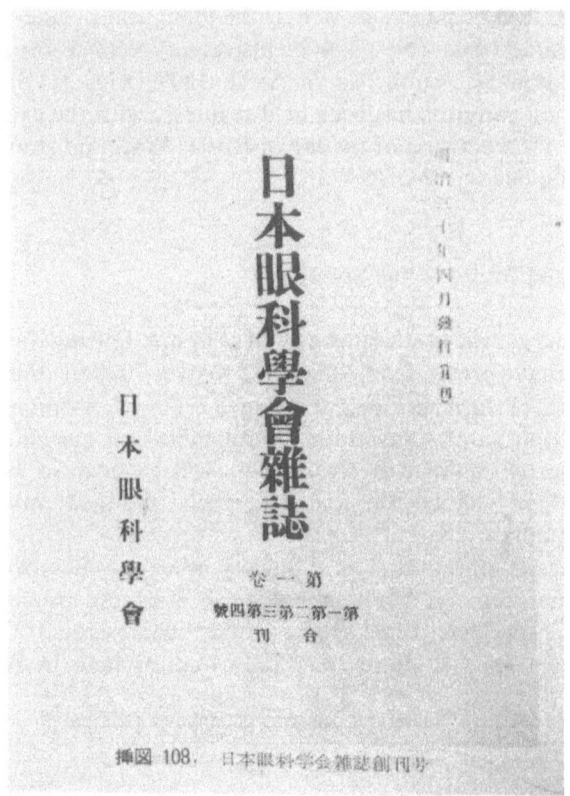

日本眼科學會雜誌

日
本
眼
科
學
會

第 一 卷

第一第二第三第四號
合 刊

挿図 108. 日本眼科学会雑誌創刊号

Fig. 4. Cover of the first issue of Acta Societatis Ophthalmologicae Japonicae, Vol. 1, Nos. 1, 2, 3 and 4, April, 1897).

hosted the 23rd International Congress in 1978 in Kyoto. It is hoped that the Japanese Ophthalmological Society will continue to serve the progress of ophthalmology in Japan as well as in the world.

References

Casey A. Wood (ed.): The American Encyclopedia and Dictionary of Ophthalmology, Cleveland Press, Chicago, 1918, Vol. XII, p. 8918.

Address for offprints: Prof. Akira Nakajima, Dept. of Ophthalmology, Juntendo School of Medicine, 3-1-3 Hongo-Bunkyo-Ku, Tokyo, Japan 113

Documenta Ophthalmologica 68: 177–184 (1988)

The general development of Chinese ophthalmology from its beginnings to the 18th century

EUGENE CHAN (1899–1986)
Zongshan Ophthalmic Center, Sun Yat-Sen University of Medical Sciences, Guangzhou, China

The infancy period of Chinese ophthalmology (1324 BC-220 AD)

Chinese medicine has a long history and there are a great number of historical records about the ancient Chinese people struggling against diseases. Some of the records are found in our oldest writings discovered in modern times. For instance, not a few diseases were mentioned in the prayers and divining words of the royal family which were engraved on the shells and bones dug out of the ruins of the Yin Dynasty – the remnants of the Wu-Ding Period (1324–1266 BC) in Anyang, Henan Province. The record of eye diseases is the earliest record of ophthalmology in our country. In the 'Hill and Sea Classic', an old book written in the period of the Qin Dynasty, more than 100 drugs are mentioned, and among them seven are related to eye diseases. Besides the 'Hill and Sea Classic' the 'Book of History', 'Book of Odes' and 'Poetry of Chu' are books recording the drugs used by our ancestors. According to the book 'Huai Nan Zi', fraxinus bungeana was beneficial to eye diseases and this kind of plant is still commonly used in Chinese medicine. Owing to the increase of the kinds of drugs and knowledge in pharmacology, a special study concerning herbs came into being. The first book on herbs in China is the 'Shen Nong Materia Medica'. It was probably completed in the Han Dynasty and is evidently a summary of the pharmacology before that time. In this book, 365 drugs including plant, animal and mineral ones were studied, those related to the eye being more than 70 – more than 40 related to promoting visual acuity and more than 30 to treating eye diseases. Some of these drugs, such as coptis chinensis and juglans mandshurica, are still valuable nowadays.

In the old books of the Qin Dynasty, one can find the character 'mu' but not the character 'yan'. It was after the Qin and Han Dynasties that the character 'yan' was gradually used. Therefore in the scripts on shells and bones eye diseases were called diseases of 'mu' instead of 'yan'.

Concerning the record of blind men, in the 'Book of History' there are such sentences as 'The blind man beat the drum' and 'The blind man made poems'. The musician Shi Kuang was a blind man. Among the famous blind men in the olden times there was 'Zi-Xia', a student of Confucius. For it was recorded in the 'Tan Gong' that 'Zi-Xia' at the age of 103 wept inconsolably over the death of his son. He subsequently lost his sight. Zuo Qiu Ming, the author of 'Spring and Autumn Annals' was also a blind man, for it was mentioned by Si Ma-Qian that 'Zuo Qiu', even though blind, wrote the book 'Guo Yu'. Judging from a line in the 'Book of Odes', blindness was classified into two categories at that time: blindness with and without pupil. Polycoria, regarding Emperor Shun (2255–2205 BC) mentioned in the 'Xun Zi' and Xiang Ji (232–202 BC), is noted in the 'Historical Records'. Both are the earliest records in the world about abnormal pupils. According to the 'Historical Records', it was said by Confucius that King Wen had farsighted eyes, and according to 'Spring and Autumn Annals' Chen Boa looked at things with his head elevated. These are probably the earliest records about errors of refraction.

The 'Canon of Internal Medicine' is an old medical book in our country, written in the period of 'Spring and Autumn'. The eye diseases mentioned in this book consist of blindness, swelling of the lower lid, jaundice of the conjunctiva, redness, pain and impairment of vision. In ophthalmology, the concept of taking the eye as a part of the whole body was stressed. In this book there is the early record of acupuncture in treatment of eye diseases. 'If redness and pain of the eyes start from the inner canthus, Yang Jiao should be taken as the needling point'. In its 'Ling Shu' section, there are such descriptions: 'The blood in 12 channel systems and 365 branches goes up to the head, and the positive spirit gets to the eye and makes the eye clear'.

In the 'Canon of Internal Medicine' the theory of the five elements (gold, wood, water, fire and earth) is also adopted. The five viscera are regarded as corresponding to five elements, and the eye is regarded as the spirit of all the viscera. So the theory of five elements was applied to ophthalmology.

In ophthalmic physiology, Guan Zi considered 'The eye comes from the "liver", and the ear from the "kidney"'. It means that during embryology the "liver" develops the eye. Pupil, cornea, conjunctiva, eye muscle, inner and outer canthus etc. are further differentiated.

The cause of eye diseases is considered due to overuse and rest for recovery is emphasized.

Besides acupuncture treatment, the ancient people knew how to treat corneal ulcer with cautery, since it is said in the old book 'Huai Nan Zi': 'The eye diseases, if not harmful to the sight, should not be cauterized'.

Once, Si Ma Shi, the Emperor, of the Jin Dynasty (265–420 AD) had a tumor in his eye and had it excised, according to the 'Book of Jin'. It was the earliest record of excising ocular tumors in our country.

Bian Que was born in the 4th century BC and was probably the earliest ophthalmologist in our country. Ophthalmologists of that time cared for patients from town to town. While passing through Luo Yang, the capital during this Zhou Dynasty, he heard that these citizens especially respected the elderly. Therefore, he decided to stay and practice there as a doctor of ear, eye and rheumatism.

Ophthalmology in the Sui-Tang Dynasties (581–907 AD)

Chinese traditional medicine in Sui-Tang Dynasties exceeded the achievements of Qin-Han Dynasties and because of interchange of medical experiences with foreign countries, it developed quickly. The earliest books on ophthalmology are 'Tao's Treatment on Eye Diseases' and 'Therapy of Eye and Ear Diseases' written by Gan Zun Zhi. Unfortunately all of them are lost.

A medical book 'General Treatise on the Causes and Symptoms of Diseases' (610 AD Chao Yuan Fang) is the earliest medical book present today on etiology and pathogenesis. It describes the causes and symptoms of diseases in more detail. According to the textual research work of the late Prof. H.T. Pi, it consists of the following: 9 eyelid diseases (blepharitis, abscess, edema and ptosis, etc.); 4 lacrimal system diseases(epiphora, xerophthalmia, chronic dacryocystitis, etc.); 7 conjunctival diseases (conjunctivitis, purulent conjunctivitis, pterygium, etc.); 4 corneal diseases (macula cornea, corneal infiltration, keratoconjunctivitis and corneal ulcers) and also the diseases of retina and optic nerve, cataract, toxemic retinopathy of pregnancy, refractive errors, strabismus and amblyopia, etc.

A famous physician Sun Si Miao (652 AD) wrote a book 'Thousand Golden Prescriptions' with copious material on preventive medicine, diagnosis, treatment and nutrition. He also observed the phenomenon of presbyopia and pointed out that the near vision of all people over 45 decreased. Besides treatment with oral drugs, he introduced the methods of irrigation, eye drops, cold and hot compress, steam and massage, as well as surgery for trachomatous pannus.

Seventy-one proven recipes for oral administration, mainly vitamins and nutrients, externally applied medicine such as coptis chinensis, fraxinus bungeana and salts, and the acupuncture points for eye diseases are included in this book.

During the Tang Dynasty, accompanying the socio-economic and cultural prosperity, international communication developed quickly. That, in turn, promoted the cultural interchange with more foreign countries. With regard to medical science, there were students coming from Korea, Japan and Arabia to study Chinese traditional medicine, while Chinese merchants, monks and priests spread Chinese medicine abroad. The famous Buddhist monk Jian Zhen had gone to Japan to teach Chinese traditional medicine. At the same time, Indian medicine was introduced into China.

In 752 AD, Wang Tao wrote 'The Medical Secrets of An Official'. In the ophthalmic parts he introduced the Indian 4 elements theory (earth, water, fire and wind) and pointed out that the eyeball consisted of 3 membranes. The causes of symptoms of cataracts and the method of couching cataracts with a metal needle were described. He had his own excellent concepts about the pathogenesis of glaucoma, considering that it was due to occlusion of eye channels, and medical treatment should be initiated as early as possible, otherwise it would become incurable.

'Eye Discussion of Long Shu' was the first famous book on ophthalmology. Unfortunately, the book was lost and the author unknown. The famous poet Bai Ju Yi who had an eye disease himself wrote a poem in which his appreciation of the book was mentioned. Originally Long Shu (later called Long Mu) was the name of a famous Indian physician in the third century AD. It was probably at that time Indian medicine was introduced into China. 'General Eye Discussion of Long Mu' still exists but it differs from the original one. It was probably written by Liu Hou in the Song Dynasty. 72 diseases are listed and were divided into two visible parts, internal and external occulopathy. The former consists of cataract, glaucoma and night blindness, and the latter consists of the diseases of cornea, conjunctiva, eyelid, lacrimal system, eye muscle, iris, trauma, trachoma, hyphema and nystagmus. In ophthalmic surgery, he introduced the operation of pterygium and stressed that excision must be complete, otherwise it might recur, the method of couching cataracts with a metal needle was mentioned.

He also introduced the theory of five wheels (water, wind, air, blood and flesh which are ophthalmologically the pupil, cornea, iris, bulbar conjunctiva and nasal-temporal canthus and eyelids) and eight walls (the intraocular structures and/or physiological functions of the eye).

In herbal medicine, Tao Hong Jink (451–563 AD) in Liang Dynasty wrote 7 volumes of 'Collective Notes to the Canon of Materia Medica'. He revised 'Shen Nong Materia Medica' and added 365 new drugs.

During the Tang Dynasty, owing to the unification of China and socioeconomic prosperity, it became necessary to revise the Chinese herbal medicine book. The Emperor Li Zhi of Tang ordered revision of the collective notes and named the revised book 'New Revised Materia Medica' which was completed in 659 AD. In it, 844 drugs were collected of which 114 were new. There were drugs coming from abroad, such as Styrax benzoiu, Piper

Nigrum, Terminalia chebula, Ferula asafoetida, etc. Some of them are used to treat eye diseases. Added by the drugs from Arabia, India and Persia, the book was more abundant in its contents and may be considered as the first pharmacopoeia in the world.

In the Tang Dynasty the imperial medical bureau was established. It was the medical education center and the medical treatment unit with many officials and students within it. Medical education range from 3–7 years according to the different specialities. There were strict examination regulations. After graduation the students might be appointed as doctors of different ranks. The five senses organ department (eye, ear, nose, throat and mouth) formerly was attached to internal medicine or surgery department, then separated as an independent department.

Enucleation was mentioned in Tang Dynasty. According to the book 'Royal Peaceful Review' 'Tsui Jia lost one eye and it was replaced by a pearl'; 'Zhou Bao' (841–846 AD) had an eye accident during a military match but emerged the victor, The Emperor awarded him a wooden eye which was technically more lifelike. These incidents, written in the 9th century, demonstrated excellent technology and the existence of ocular surgery even at that early time.

Ophthalmology in the Song-Jin-Yuan Dynasties (960–1368 AD)

Wang Huei Yin (978–992 AD) et al. edited 'Holy Peaceful Benevolent Prescriptions', which represented the prescriptions and proven recipes extant before the Song Dynasty and discussed the etiology and pathogenesis of diseases. It consisted of 2 volumes, medical and surgical ophthalmology. In medical ophthalmology, he introduced and summarized the five-wheels-theory and stressed preventive medicine and nutrition. In surgical ophthalmology, he introduced the procedures of excision, hook, acupuncture etc. Cataract extraction was discussed especially in greater detail, such as preoperative precautions and postoperative treatment. He also discussed the treatment of bleeding, pain, vomiting, etc. This classic constitutes valuable ophthalmic literature.

During about the 11th century, 'Holy Review of Recipes' was published, in which proven and imperial recipes were also collected. There are 12 volumes in ophthalmology. 758 recipes are related to eye diseases and a method of making pills of immortality was described. Emperor Zhao Zhe was captured in battle and was noted to be blind in one eye. This blindness was attributed to toxicity from the pills of immortality which is now known to contain mercury.

In the Song Dynasty, owing to the import of drugs from Arabia, Southeast Asia as well as the newly found herbs in China, the old materia medica was not sufficient, so it was revised many times. One of the most important achievements in the Song Dynasty was the publication of 'Revised Materia Medica', written Tang Shen Wei. Later it was revised twice by the officials of the imperial medical bureau. Finally it was combined with another book 'Amplification on Canon of Materia Medica' by Kou Zong Shi. The combined book consists of 30 volumes, including 1740 different drugs of which 180 are related to eye diseases. It is a complete pharmacopoeia and regarded as the standard book for nearly 500 years.

'Essentials of Ophthalmology' was published after the Song Dynasty and according to the reasearch work of Kokawa, the author was Tien Ren Zhai. The theory of five wheels and eight walls as well as the basic principle of surface and interior, sthenia and asthenia, and the relationship between eye and general system were discussed. Oral medications accompanied by external therapy was stressed and 80 eye diseases were listed, their symptoms, causes and treatment together with a brief atlas. Special attention was paid to the examination of pupil, cornea, iris, bulbar and palpebral conjunctiva. The operations for entropion and couching with a metal needle were introduced.

The imperial medical bureau consisted of nine separate branches in the Song Dynasty. Thus, ophthalmology was first established as an independent department.

During the Song Yuan Dynasties, many schools of thought among physicians appeared. Each one brought forth new concepts of his own. Finally, four schools of medical thought developed as follows:

1. Fire-heat theory   Liu Wan Su (1110–1200 AD)
2. Purgation theory   Zhang Cong Zhen (1156–1228 AD)
3. Spleen and stomach theory   Li Gao (1180–1251 AD)
4. Nourish Yin theory   Zhu Zhen Heng (1281–1358 AD)

All of them had their own characteristics but consisted of the same principle of treatment based on differentiation of symptoms and signs.

Spectacles were mentioned as early as the Song Dynasty, a judicial officer Shih Hong wore a crystal glass to improve his vision. This might be the first record of using spectacles. A more reliable record was mentioned in a book called 'Dong Tien Qing Lu' written by Zhao Hsi Hou – an imperial clansman in South Song Dynasty. 'Ai Dai can help the old to read small words and if without it, the old cannot see to read'. Ai Dai are ancient words for spectacles. In the Ming Dynasty (1368–1644 AD) Ai Dai was mentioned in several records, such as 'Ai Dai is as large as a coin with the colour of mica. It can improve the poor vision of old.' 'The noblemen have spectacles.' during Qing Dynasty the word 'spectacles' was used more popularly.

Ophthalmology in the Ming-Qing Dynasties (1368–1911 AD)

The famous ophthalmologist Ni Wei De (1303–1377 AD) wrote the book 'Causes and Mechanisms of Eye Diseases' published in 1372 AD, which consisted of 2 volumes. The etiology and classification of diseases, divided into 18 different groups are described in the first volumes. Treatment consists of a combination of 20–30 herbs. Wei De stressed that there is in each packet a main ingredient called 'Monarch' and the lesser ingredients are called 'Minister', 'Assistant', and 'Guide' in decreasing order of importance. 18 different kinds of diseases are listed as follows: diseases of eye lid, lacrymal system, conjunctiva, cornea, iris, lens, primary and traumatic glaucoma, night blindness, trauma and nutritional deficiency, etc. Ni had abundant clinical experiences and carried out excellent pathological (pathogenesis) research work. He classified the etiology clearly and developed his own concepts.

Another author Wang Keng Tang (1602 AD) wrote a book 'Standards of Diagnosis and treatment of Six Categories of Diseases'. It is a book of clinical treatment and diagnosis in which the symptoms and causes are discussed thoroughly with prescriptions included. In 1644 AD, Fu Ren Yu edited 'A Precious Book of Ophthalmology'. It is an ophthalmic book consisting of 6 volumes. In volume 1, there is general discussion. In volume 2, the afore-mentioned theories of etiologies, and in volumes 3–6, 108 kinds of eye diseases with an atlas of acupuncture points and prescriptions at the end. Fu stressed ophthalmic surgery, but he suggested that it be performed cautiously. In the Ming Dynasty there was a book 'Private Copy of Complete Book on Ophthalmology' edited by Ai Xui Yuan. All the aforementioned theories and also the list of 72 diseases with atlas and characters of Chinese herbs are mentioned.

In Ming Dynasty Zhu Hsiao wrote 'Prescriptions for Curing All People' which is the most complete prescription book up to present days, consisting of 168 volumes and 61,000 prescriptions.

During the 16th century, the great pharmacologist Li Shih Zhen (1518–1593 AD), wrote a world famous book 'Compendium of Materia Medica'. There were 52 volumes listing 1892 drugs of which 374 were new. There were

184

420 related to ophthalmology, 120 for improving vision and 300 for treatment. Later, Zhao Xue Min (1765 AD) in Qing Dynasty wrote 'Supplement of compendium of materia Medica'.

During Qing Dynasty there were even more books on medication for ophthalmology books: 3 volumes of 'Complete Book on Ophthalmology' by Huang Ting Jing, 'Zhang's Medicine' by Zhang Lu, 'Golden Mirror for Original Medicine' by Wu Qian, etc.

The Imperial Medical Bureau was expanded from nine to thirteen branches in the Ming Dynasty. Ophthalmology was again independent and there now were physicians who only practiced ophthalmology. Although the Medical Bureau was reduced to eleven branches in the Qing Dynasty, ophthalmology still remained one of them.

According to the research work of Suzuki paracentesis was initially performed at the beginning of the Ming Dynasty (1377 AD) in China, however Hirschberg and Suzuki stated that it was at the end of Ming Dynasty. The British ophthalmologist Touberville, following the Chinese method, applied paracentesis of sclera in 17th century.

Address for offprints: Zongshan Ophthalmic Center, Sun Yat-Sen University of Medical Sciences, Guangzhou, China